Dying Words

Dying
Words

TALKING POINTS FOR MORTALS

Susan E. Sheehan
Lake Forest, Illinois

ISBN: 1505253160
ISBN 13: 9781505253160

for
Dennis Patrick Sheehan, who showed me my voice and gave me reason to use it, and the Other Wife who does not yet know the language

CHAPTER 1

Etiology

[ee-tee-ol-uh-jee] n. the philosophical study of the origins of disorder; from the Greek for "give a reason why"

Lying beside my husband's hospital bed in the intensive care unit with only a sheet between me and the frighteningly septic tile floor, I have the sleepless hours of the night to think. My mind wanders. Somewhere along the way, I pick up a companion. I call her the "Other Wife." She's a waitress or teacher or accountant who, like me, is watching as her husband's life slips away before her eyes. But unlike me, she doesn't have a background in medical social work. She's not familiar with the varied and at times strange subcultures within hospitals: emergency departments' mixes of the mundane and macabre, medical-surgical floors' mapped-out methods and rigid routines, operating rooms' soundtracks (from classical to heavy metal, depending on the surgeons' taste) blaring, only to be out-chimed by the ICU's many monitors—both human and machine.

How do you, precious Other Wife, absorb the sights and sounds of this alien space?

It occurs to me that even if she can muster up the courage to ignore the nurses' post-visiting-hours glares, the Other Wife probably has no idea how to advocate for her husband in his time of great need. A wave of compassion rises up in me as I can only imagine what it would be like to be so utterly ill equipped for this daunting task.

The Other Wife clings to me as I move through the last ten days of Dennis's life. At first I would like to shake her off. She's distracting me. I tell myself I should focus on my reason for lying on that floor of the ICU. The man I adore is dying. But nobody knows how long this process of dying will take—somewhere in the days-to-years range, I'm told. There's also disagreement around the etiology of Dennis's ragged decline.

Do you understand the etiology of your husband's disease, Other Wife? Do you even know what that means?

Words like "etiology" are part of my workplace lexicon. Remember, I began spending my days (and many nights) in hospitals and hospice settings long before my husband fell ill. Passionate as I am about medical social work, I never could have imagined the intensely personal value my expanded vocabulary would accrue. The lack of clarity surrounding the origins of Dennis's disease, as you might expect, led to a proportionate lack of consensus around what interventions this large, urban teaching hospital might offer him. That's why I'm here. I want to be sure the hospital acts in Dennis's best interest at all times. He and I have discussed his wishes, and I'm generally clear about what I need to do for him.

But I imagine you, Other Wife, are less sure. Oh, honestly, how could you not be? I speak the language of this place, and I'm barely able to do what I'm here to do.

Within a couple of hours of meeting her, my mind shares its corridors with the Other Wife, and we make peace. Although I wonder at times if insanity awaits around the next bend, I come to realize that this inward, imaginary relationship is not so much a matter of my own benevolence, but is born of mutual needs, if you will. Thinking of the Other Wife serves me well as Dennis's dramatic decline relegates me to ever-increasingly bizarre psychosocial spaces. She keeps me company. She gives my experience context. Yes, she requires some attention that I might apply elsewhere as my marriage unravels in that hospital bed, but she becomes my invisible cohort as I interact with the chief medical officer, the director of quality services, and various medical doctors who tend to Dennis in his final days.

You, dear Other Wife, give me a purpose larger than my loss. And my loss is staggering.

Nobody would ask the age-old question "Death, where is thy sting?" if indeed the two—death and sting—were not inexorably linked. Nobody even wants to mention the *D* word, yet our collective code of silence only amplifies the proverbial sting. Americans whisper and hush their talk of death as if speaking openly will somehow bring it on. But you don't need a medical degree to know that, ultimately, death can't be averted. While poignant and wrenching, dying, like all of life, presents precious gifts to those who are willing and able to engage in the process.

As varied as it is universal, death in twenty-first-century America is no simple matter. With medical technology advancing by leaps and bounds, life expectancy has climbed faster than the US health care system can recalibrate. Bioethics and end-of-life issues have become the stuff of national discourse, local news, and family history. People are far more likely to receive long-term treatment for chronic illnesses like diabetes and heart disease or to be buoyed by joint replacements and cardiac stent implants than they are to die from a sudden heart attack or out-of-the-blue lethal pneumonia. Now more than ever, Americans need to know the language required to navigate dying as a process rather than as a single event. The demand for a new vocabulary is apparent to anyone who would like to exercise some modicum of control over their own dying days or those of their loved ones. Albeit tenuous, this sense of control can actually steady the hand that reaches for meaning both within and beyond the loss.

Most of us started asking questions about death around our second birthdays. Inquisitive toddlers and adults alike, myself included, almost always begin and end with an array of "whys" when pondering questions surrounding death. I have always held far more questions than answers. The questions occasionally offer an answer or two but more often act as vectors to yet more questions. So it's only fair to begin with a confession: I don't have very many answers. Worse, I confess this with no apology. After all, who among us has found much in life to be what we had imagined? Rather than searching endlessly for life's elusive answers, we must learn to live in the questions. This is not to say that I've given up on asking the tough questions. Quite the contrary. Formulating questions focuses our attention. Like a reporter, we instinctively ask, "Who, what, when, where, why, and how?" We gather data. We decide what we can let go, and we wrestle with what we cannot. We formulate conclusions. Sitting with our questions broadens our sense of self and solidifies our place in this world. Sharing our questions builds our sense of community. And if we should stumble upon an answer somewhere in this process, all the better.

My guess is that those who avoid the questions are no more enlightened but rather more disenchanted than the rest of us. They simply gave in to the temptation to give up. Somehow, in this era of mass communications and seemingly endless information, it seems we should understand more about life and death than we do. But in the dark of the night, the existential questions of the ages float like cartoon ghosts around us. Who am I? Where have I been? Where am I going? What is the meaning of life? Is this all there is? What should I be doing with my life? For those of us distracted by health care and medical ethics, other questions reverberate. Are we really healthier because of evolving technologies? When is life support an appropriate option? Do the poor receive the same quality of care as the rich? How should the answers to these questions influence medical care, conceptually, and end-of-life care, practically? These are big questions that coalesce until their ghosts blitz our night ceilings white. It's the seemingly little questions, however, that threaten to darken those ceilings again. What happens when this life ends? How will I die? How will the people I love die? What can I do about it? *Should* I do those things? Is it okay to admit being unprepared and frightened?

I know you're scared, Other Wife. So am I...So am I.

Nothing brings these questions to our attention like impending death. And as much as death leaves in its wake deep loss, dying itself can be a process as vital as any other part of life. Thinking gets focused. Priorities are ordered. Relationships gain clarity. And the hard questions surface. Even if these questions have no answers, their formulation helps make meaning out of what our culture seems to have denied: dying is part of life. All of life, regardless of the circumstances, personalities, and details, can be done well. But it is impossible to die well without asking the questions. Not without grappling with the tensions. And not without speaking the language that allows us to ask and grapple.

Dying Words tells the story of my husband's last ten days on earth. My Dennis was a statistical outlier. His disease progression, exacerbated by a constellation of pain syndromes, could not have been modified or ameliorated even if it had been better understood. And it was not at all well understood. That Dennis had a progressive disease was thoroughly documented, even though the extent of his physical suffering was not consistently noted. His excruciating pain did not respond to steroids or opiates variously administered. Alternative therapies were tried with no effect. Spinal stimulation, bariatric chambers, acupuncture, mind-body interventions, dietary therapies, and almost constant prayer did not fend off the nightmarish parade of symptoms assaulting his body.

All of this was history by the time we entered the hospital that final time, but because Dennis presented so differently than the typical patient, he was deemed an inappropriate candidate for some elements of end-of-life care. And as I alluded to earlier, countless inconclusive conversations regarding his disease's etiology—how it originated and progressed—fed controversy among his medical team. My role was to stand in the space between these skilled professionals and navigate the best possible course for this man on whom my personal sun really did rise and set.

In the midst of this chaos, I could still see the facts as they presented themselves to me. First and foremost, Dennis was a remarkable man. His courage, grace, and indefatigable will to live life to its fullest at times disguised the seriousness of his disease and its fatal trajectory. He was ultimately trapped in a body racked with unremitting and ultimately truly unbearable pain. It was my duty and privilege to serve as his advocate during this final hospitalization.

During that ten-day period, Dennis came to personify the tension between two polar opposites within the US health care system: traditional medicine, with its primary goal of keeping people alive, and palliative medicine, with its mission to support dying people and their families. Fortunately, I was in familiar territory, as my daily workplaces included both ICU and hospice settings.

I was able to take time away from my regular job in order to concentrate on Dennis 24/7 when he entered the hospital—but this was anything but a postman's holiday. As our twenty-fifth wedding anniversary approached, we were privileged to be passionately in love and deeply committed to one another. Dennis was the patient, which meant that the medical care plan and the questions around care and preferences were directed at him, theoretically. But in fact, more than at any other time in adult life, as death approaches the term "patient system" applies more and more. Typically, at the end of life, loved ones gather and of necessity become increasingly active in the patient's experience. They start out ordering the meals. Then they move the dishes closer. And finally, they spoon the food into mouths that will be ingesting less and less. As the patient's physical and mental faculties decline, a host of needs arise. A vanguard is needed. An advocate. A voice. A sidekick, should there be any light moments. That I was prepared to articulate what Dennis could no longer assert for himself was indeed a severe mercy. I would have wrested that privilege from him sooner had I been granted the opportunity, but in truth, it's the hardest job I've ever had.

Are you willing to step up to this job, Other Wife? I know you don't want to face the reality that your husband may soon die, and believe me, nobody is ever prepared for the dreaded tasks and decisions associated with death and dying. But your husband needs your help. He needs a champion, now more than ever.

Dying Words is for the Other Wives—and husbands, family members, and friends—who must come alongside their dying loved ones and walk with them to the threshold of this life. It is my honor to serve as a docent of sorts to others who follow the path Dennis and I traveled together. Though I already spoke the language of modem medicine when I took on this job, the mythical Other Wife does not. So, I'm committed to holding her hand and leading her through the maze of end-of-life care in the US health care system. More than that, I'd like to embrace her and tell her how important I know her newfound and totally unwanted job is. The Other Wife and I stand side by side in solidarity. She's just now coming to understand her role and she has a lot of valid—even haunting—questions. She and I dialogue at odd hours about topics most people don't want to broach. We abandon modesty and social convention for the greater goal of sharing this bizarre space between our real worlds and the day we will go home as widows.

Picture her as I did from the first night we met in the ICU where Dennis lay dying. The Other Wife is middle-aged, but her visage and carriage reflect years of hardship.

Her family ekes out a living wage, but their health insurance is lousy. She has nagging physical issues of her own. This day is focused on her husband, but she can't afford to miss another day of work. She calls the hospital on her break, but the RN assigned to her husband is busy with patient care and doesn't return the call in the narrow window allotted. The Other Wife goes directly to the hospital after work, but the express bus is full, and she has to ride the local. She rushes to her husband's hospital room but then hesitates. She slowly approaches the bed, tentatively leans over him, and kisses his forehead. He doesn't respond. She stands back and thinks twice before gently touching his hand. She surveys all of the monitors and lines and bags that surround his bed and wonders if anything has changed since the day before.

She knows her husband's primary care physician's name, but she hasn't seen him during this hospitalization. "Why is he never here?" she wonders. None of the drugs being administered are familiar to her. All those multisyllabic interventions batted back and forth leave her feeling like she's losing a game of monkey in the middle. Hospital jargon floats past her because nothing in her life experience thus far anchors it. All of the people in pastel scrubs look the same to her—nurses, orderlies, technicians. She's never quite sure with whom she's talking. One of these hospital professionals comes in and asks the Other Wife if she has any questions. She shakes her head, although she has dozens. The nurse scratches a note in the chart stating "spouse seems unaware of prognosis," hands the pen to the Other Wife, and asks her to sign consents. The Other Wife signs without hesitation so that the doctors can help her husband. She trusts them to do what is best.

The Other Wife breaks free from this alien culture to connect with her husband in a more familiar language. She has brought his favorite ice cream. He's too tired to take more than the bit she gingerly places on his lips. She tries to tell him about her day, but his eyes travel to a point behind her. Then they close again. She slouches in the squeaky plastic chair and stares at her husband's face. It is puffy, ashen, and needing a shave. She's not accustomed to the overgrowth. In contrast to yesterday's shivering, the sweat on his temples catches and holds the glow from the fluorescent lighting. The RN comes in and greets the Other Wife cheerfully before busying herself taking vitals, tinkering with what she calls the "smart pump," and questioning aloud how long the IV in his forearm has been there. The date written on the tape holding the line steady is smudged.

"He's been here for a week," the Other Wife reports. "But I don't know how long that's been in his arm. Is it bad to leave it in too long?"

"We like to change the lines every three days to prevent infection," the RN explains. "But if it's patent, I don't really want to mess with it."

The Other Wife doesn't understand the answer to the single, measly question she was bold enough to ask. Her biggest questions don't seem sophisticated enough to pose: Is he getting better or worse? Why isn't he eating much? When can he come home? Abject fear prevents her from asking questions like, How am I going to take care of him when he comes home? Family is scattered and resources are scarce. The Other Wife has no plan for caring for a gravely ill man if her insurance company decides his "eligible days" at the hospital are up. She has heard that happens to people without warning. Or even worse, what if he never comes home? Her worry is interrupted by the crackle of the intercom speaker followed by a dispassionate voice announcing, for the third and final time, that visiting hours are over.

Remember, Other Wife, this is your husband and he needs you. You have every right to be here.

Dennis's story encapsulates both what can go terribly wrong at the end of life and what can be sublimely right. The difference is in large part a function of the relationship between the patient system and the medical team. Does the medical team regard the patient as a Saint-Exupery "unique in all the world" person or merely a cluster of symptoms? Is the patient palliated or parsed? Does the average American know the difference? The more you know about end-of-life care, the better your chances of securing appropriate measures for yourself or your loved ones.

The palliative service officially admitted Dennis for hospital care in light of his severe and intractable pain. On the palliative care floor, all of the MDs and ancillary members of the team use their first names with patients. They come to Dennis's room multiple times each day and sit at Dennis's bedside as they examine him, presumably to communicate their willingness to prioritize him (and me as his wife) by meeting him at his eye level. Their posture communicates to us that they are fully present during their time in Dennis's room. As they move past me in this crowded space, they always seem to steady me with a hand on my knee or an arm brushed across my shoulder. They ask me questions about Dennis's condition and really seem to value my answers. They ask repeatedly how I'm coping.

The medical department under which Dennis's diagnosis falls also participates in his care during his final hospital stay. For the most part, their care is professionally competent. That said, it contrasts markedly with the palliative service. Specialists from various medical disciplines occasionally barge through the door as if they have some degree of ownership in Dennis's case. These dispassionate doctors don't bring any interdisciplinary team members with them. They don't come often, nor do they stay long. They see no reason to sit. Reluctant to touch Dennis, these MDs never think to inquire about my well-being. Their clinical attention focuses on the manifestations of Dennis's nightmarish disease course, which moves so quickly that its progression can be measured in hours. When asked directly, these MDs offer me their opinions, but they never ask for my input on anything and generally discourage dialogue of any kind. This scenario may not be typical of all hospital experiences, but it surely isn't unusual.

Before I go further, I must offer a few caveats. Each person depicted in this story would likely write about their role differently than I do, and I speak only from my own experience of our intersections. But the story wouldn't be complete without the full cast of characters. With regard to the many health care professionals involved, some medical specialties and all professional names have been changed in the interest of discretion, but the people described are neither fictitious nor composites. Dialogue is reconstructed from memory with every reasonable attempt to render it true in essence, if not verbatim. In print, I never ascribe motives to the actions I witnessed, although I realize that in my head and yours such leaps are inevitable. While aspects of Dennis's physical situation are described in great detail in an attempt to broaden the implications of his story and minimize minutia, his actual disease is not revealed.

You would rightfully suspect that I can't pretend to be dispassionate in flattening my husband's last ten days onto these pages like a faded bloom pressed between the pages of a book. It might help you to know that I make no attempt. I'm open—even eager—for you to take what is my story and weave it with yours. Our discrete threads are part of the warp and weft of a larger tapestry of innumerable personal experiences on the loom of the US health care system.

This book deals specifically with issues of end-of-life health care, although the nature of the subject makes it difficult to know exactly where we are on its course at any given time. Death can be predictable, but it more often holds the element of surprise. Other times it evades all expectations. I can't offer much advice as to how to make peace with this uncertainty, but I can attest to the importance of preparing for death in such a way that you are part of its process rather than simply one of its casualties.

Dying well is contingent in part on good science: pain management, catheterization, alternating pressure mattresses, anti-anxiety interventions, and a vast array of pharmacological treatments. But the protocol should not begin and end with raw science. Dying well can be made breathtakingly beautiful by the overlay of creative arts and medicine. Personal affections and affinities and accommodations can make all the difference in the world as people straddle that place between life and death. I have a dream that someday science and art will cooperate rather than compete within the US health care system. Between now and then, we must share our stories and work for a better end-of-life ethos in America.

My husband was an exceptional man, and in some ways his story is exceptional. But in other ways, the end-of-life story is universal. The mystery surrounding the disease that took Dennis's life makes his case unusual (it would ultimately require an extensive autopsy to begin to understand what Dennis suffered). But even as scientific progress marches forward, mystery remains an integral element of modem medicine. Indeed, Dennis's story would be dramatic as an isolated occurrence, but its telling is more imperative because it is, in reality, fairly common. While our society shuts up the secrets of death in the sterile recesses of the medical world—much to the detriment of all who must eventually experience life's one true reality—I want to reach out and guide. Take my hand.

TALKING POINTS FOR MORTALS

1. Are there treatments that you do not understand? Are there treatments that you do not want?
2. What is your greatest concern around the medical history of any presenting symptoms? How are you thinking that this concern might be addressed?

■ ■ ■

CHAPTER 2

Faith

[feyth] n. a (1): belief and trust in and loyalty to God, (2): belief in the traditional doctrines of a religion;
b (1): firm belief in something for which there is no proof, (2): complete trust

Join with me in remembering Dennis's final trip to the hospital. Unlike everything else about our situation, the weather is perfect on this midsummer day. It might surprise you that Dennis elects to ride the train to the city hospital on the last day he ever wears street clothes. His reasoning? He can neither sit nor stand nor crouch nor crawl for more than a few minutes at a time. Riding in a car is sheer torture for him. On the train you can stand, sit, move around, and basically do whatever you want. People may look at you askance, but if you're sick enough you stop noticing. Life becomes about surviving each step with enough courage leftover to take the one after that. Your world becomes astoundingly small.

But how is it that as Dennis's world shrinks before our eyes, his faith seems to grow inversely? His is the type of faith that fits the definition "complete trust" unequivocally. Friends, family, and perfect strangers see Dennis's faith in action as he somehow finds the grace to deal with the losses and suffering wrought by treacherous disease without harboring any bitterness, self-pity, or guile toward anyone. Dennis doesn't hide the reality of his situation, but he refuses to pass his affliction on to the ones he loves. He wants to be a blessing and not a burden, perhaps as much because of his illness as in spite of it.

Over the course of his final hospitalization, the fact that Dennis walks into the hospital becomes a point of confusion. How could anyone with an advanced, progressive disease *walk* into his last week of life? Well, for the record, it is worth adjusting the focus of the picture. Erase the image of Dennis walking in as a basically strong, middle-aged man with a classy walking stick. His steps are not strides as much as spastic lurches. His gait is tentative and irregular. Sometimes his steps are lengthened by lack of control, and other times they are shortened by fear of that same lack of control. First Dennis slides his braced right leg to meet his left. Then he leans forward, his gaze fixed on his cane about two feet in front of him. Dennis focuses on that cane like a *drishti*, a technique he learned from the yoga lessons he's taking, in hopes of slowing the freefall decline in strength and flexibility he's experiencing. Focusing on a *drishti* is supposed to bring better balance, but this Sanskrit word also means *vision*, *intelligence*, or *wisdom*. Dennis plumbs all of these sources of strength just to get from point A to point

B. The cane, usually held in his right hand unless sore elbows and shoulders demand he use his left, thrusts forward. His body bends over; his weight spills onto the grip of the cane just under his ribs. He attempts to straighten up, or at least partially unfold, on this last lurch forward. Then he repeats the arduous process again. Step after step, day after day, he dances his painful, awkward dance.

Dennis is clearly largely spent by the travel when we arrive at the hospital. He is patient during the ninety minutes we wait in the lobby with his suitcase. Usually talkative, he says very little. He is restless and suffering gravely over the next few hours when he and two other patients, coupled with their respective baggage handlers, are ushered to basement recliners. After a few hours, the RN sitting at the desk notices Dennis's visible discomfort and offers him a Tylenol. Normally, he would have had something witty to say about such an absurd offer, likening it to giving an umbrella to someone caught in a cyclone or something like that. But now Dennis just politely declines. The RN, sensing the awkwardness of the moment, fumbles with her paperwork nervously as her eyes follow Dennis's gyrations up, down, and around his assigned recliner. There is no way he can just settle into it and nap, which is apparently the intent. When a room on the floor finally opens up, Dennis is the first to be escorted to it.

My husband is greatly diminished by his illness, but he remains at his core gracious, compassionate, and socially engaging. He continues to tell great stories. He loves an audience. That works well for him since he usually has one. I, being more introverted by nature, have always relished the quieter times as we simply go about the business of living life together. Those times have been fewer and further between as we lead up to this hospitalization. Dennis's disease is so crippling that I have come to refer to it as an unwelcome guest who has taken up residence in the midst of our marriage. I don't blame Dennis for being distracted by the incessant demands of this interloper, but I never do make peace with her. A few months earlier, in a moment of exasperation, I blurted out,

"Your disease doesn't trump everything!" I may have been right theoretically, but practically, Dennis and I both knew I was wrong. He just stared at me.

While Dennis describes every detail of the impact of his disease on his body, he is remarkably brave in the face of unthinkable pain. So much so that his listeners tend to miss the point of his description. I've often described him as a mensch firmly rooted in an Irish Catholic heritage. His stoic nature, coupled with his upbringing in an athletic family of nine, imbued in him a "no pain, no gain" mentality in which whining is not an option. As a result, it's virtually impossible for Dennis to advocate for himself when he's sick. So, during a comprehensive admissions process at a major US teaching hospital, my extremely articulate husband is unable to say the words that need—in my considered opinion—to be said.

Every waking moment is excruciating. Dennis vacillates between being sure that he is dying and being terrified that perhaps he is not. We're first in line for this coveted admission because I told an MD whom I trust that, in my work in ICUs and in hospice, I have never seen anyone so miserably uncomfortable as Dennis. My anxiety is palpable. Dr. Anna Peters believes me and greases the skids for us by calling a palliative care colleague late on a Friday afternoon. Dr. Daniel Hayes follows by making the necessary arrangements for a Monday admission.

Now it is that Monday. Dennis's pain is beyond unbearable, and we need help. This is my husband's chance to present the crazy catalogue of symptoms that inhabit his body and engage some of the sharpest minds in the country to alleviate his pain, if only for a limited time. It's a long shot, but we're desperate. I listen as quietly as I possibly can through each interview. First, Dennis is examined and questioned by an advanced practice nurse (APN) named Jane Marsh, while a registered nurse (RN) places an IV line in his left hand in order to record what might be objectively assessed in Dennis's mysterious decline. Jane is gentle and direct. Her eyes narrow in periodically in resonance with aspects of Dennis's struggle. Her measured manner is calming. She is young, but she carries herself like a seasoned professional. I try to rest in my observation of the familiar hospital routine. I tell myself that some of the anxiety I feel is just my own drama around the serious illness that is robbing me of my husband. I will myself to stop fidgeting and focus on the people rotating in and out of the room with its waterfront view of the city skyline.

Jane leaves for a time and then returns with the palliative care physician working on the inpatient unit that week, Dr. Kara Linstra. Dr. Kara's compact frame winds through the crowded room like a drop of rain sliding down a window pane. She has the sort of energy that tells me she is seated only to graciously meet her new patient at eye level and not because of any need to get off her feet. She and Jane work well as a team. We draw from them a sense of peace that comes from the possibility that there are indeed people who are committed to doing whatever they can to give Dennis some relief. I take a deep breath and try again to train my mind on these gracious caregivers. But instead I find myself wondering if our daughters will remember to walk the dog.

The palliative service is generous with their attention to Dennis. They don't rush. I know their time is precious, but they conduct this intake process as if they have nothing else to do on this particular afternoon. My goal is to be sure that they understand how terribly sick my Dennis has come to be. He, as usual, presents as perfectly charming. He knows every detail of the illness attacking his body. He lives with it every day. But in a room with an audience, Dennis acts like—well, like Dennis. He answers each question like a reporter on location, suppressing all signs of the angst and agony he's feeling. He leaves out the part about stuffing his mouth with a towel and biting down with all of his might to stifle pain-sparked screams. He talks about being able to manage activities of daily living (ADLs) but doesn't reveal that they consume the entire day. He doesn't tell Jane and Dr. Kara that he no longer uses a knife or scissors because he can't direct their blades. He doesn't mention that he often chokes on food and more often on liquids but refuses to use a thickener because, in his estimation, he's "not at that stage yet." Dennis is charming when we need tragic.

I'm anything but charming. I'm edgy. I interrupt frequently. I clarify details when no one asks for my input. I am
not even a little bit amused by the easy joking and social
pleasantries with which Dennis punctuates his medical history. I'm determined to tell this new team of professionals exactly what they're up against. I suspect some of them
think I have an agenda. They're right. I'm committed to securing whatever help might be available for the man whom
I have seen choking on his tears, begging God to give him
the grace to cope minute by minute. While Dennis employs
the handsome, dimpled smile that has served him well his
entire life, I see past it to the pain-rendered frown lines that
have forged a new and complex topography on my fifty-
two-year-old husband's face.

Periodically Dennis and I are alone in the room for brief
breaks in the assessment process. My frustration thickens
the air. I want to be gentle and affirming, but I'm convinced
that Dennis's charm is undermining his own case.

"You won't get the best care if you sanitize everything,"
I try to explain.

"I *am* telling them everything," Dennis replies, surprised
by my chiding.

"You're describing symptoms like you're one of the clinicians. There's no urgency in your voice. You need to let
them know how desperate you are!"

"I don't need to be melodramatic."

"Yes, you do! Every time you aren't, you leave it to me
to make your case, and I resent being forced to sound like a
heavy-handed bitch."

"That's your choice." He shrugs and asks me to help him traverse the four feet to the bathroom.

"You didn't tell them you had trouble getting to the bathroom," I can't keep from shooting as he leans heavily on my shoulders. With my words ringing as a challenge, Dennis tries to straighten up on his own, but he doesn't have the strength. Being vindicated doesn't make me feel any better.

Dennis is tired and really doesn't have it in him to deal with my criticism. I feel guilty. But more, I feel anxious that he might not get the care he needs, as has been the case on and off for the last three years. Finally, he states the obvious: "You don't have to stay. You're not helping me. You should go home and come back tomorrow."

"Not helping you? I got Dr. Peters to call the palliative team and Dr. Lucy to examine you at home, and I've done all your paperwork and given half of your history!" I fume. Keenly aware of the fact that I've become a net emotional drain on the situation, I'm ashamed of losing my self-control and of contributing to Dennis's discomfort in any way at all. I pick up a novel in an attempt to recalibrate, but I can't help stealing glances at my husband struggling to change from his street clothes to hospital garb. I want so much to be the perfect wife for this man I adore, but his disease had taken its toll on me as surely as it has chipped away at him. I have a headache.

By the time the June sky has darkened, we're holding our irritation with each other better. Holding it, but not entirely resolving it. I'm grateful that our relationship remains honest and real through it all, but I have no way of knowing that this day will be Dennis's last fully conversational one.

It's only in retrospect that I see the swollen significance of each day. Eventually, I kiss Dennis and head for the commuter train. Soon after the stale, dimly lit train pulls out of the station, my cell phone rings. Dennis wants to be sure we are okay. We recommit ourselves to one another and to doing all of life together with love and respect. We both ask forgiveness and readily grant it. As has so often been the case, it seems that we are ending our day closer than if we had never fought in the first place. We talk of our abiding love and unconditional commitment to one another as I ride north. It's sappy. It's wonderful.

I call Dennis again later to say goodnight. He sounds on the verge of panic. His bowels and bladder are spastic, so he isn't able to rest. His core strength seems appreciably weaker than it was just a few hours before. He tells me that, earlier, he fell near his bed and wasn't able to get up until someone heard him calling out and came to help him. He's become a "two-person assist." I tell him I'm coming back to the hospital right away, but he says he's going to try to sleep and asks if I'll come early in the morning. I agree to go with our original plan and pray for some rest before I head back to my husband's bedside.

Dennis calls a number of times during the night to ask me to bring him things in the morning. He wants the Invisalign braces he wears on his teeth at night. Even as the rest of his body is racked with pain, he's thinking about his teeth. I see the irony in this request, but I validate its importance as Dennis grasps for fragments of the routine that once ordered his life. He also wants the *New York Times*, another predictable, comforting request. And then, close to midnight, he calls because he wants me to bring him the rolling walker. He thinks that he has lost the strength needed to manage the intricate choreography of two weak, spastic legs and one cane. In this last request there is no comfort. But I have a renewed commitment to serve this man, whose voice reveals a profound vulnerability, in any way I can.

At dawn's first light, I load the car with all of Dennis's requested props. I want to bring him something special as well. I want to remind him that I'm in this battle with him. I want to assuage my guilt over the previous day's interaction. So, before I leave the house, I draw him a picture. No flowers or hearts here; it's a graph. I use a thick, black marker to sketch a normal bell curve with an elongated right tail. I draw a star beyond the tail where it merges with the x-axis and label that spot dm (short for "Dream Man," my private nickname for this man who really is the stuff of my dreams.) I want to show him that he's well beyond the curve, beyond excellent in every way. I want to remind him of my conviction of that truth for as long as he holds the cognitive capacity to appreciate it. I think it will be a good reminder for me, too, should Dennis and I have another lapse into the land of what I have come to think of as my "marriage to other people's husbands". Those are the times when he acts in ways that make me hold back the "Dream" part of his nickname—when he's selfish or critical or insensitive to my feelings. Or should I say, "tender little feelings," which was how he and his four brothers derided all things emotional when they were teenagers. In some cases, those tender little feelings are mine. Still, on this morning I am keenly aware that our marriage is grinding to a halt, and I want us both to feel safe in it. Safe in each other.

Finding a convenient parking spot is easy at six thirty in the morning. I drape our various supplies around the rolling walker and push it across the parking garage, looking like a bag lady heading west. I find Dennis asleep in the shrouded room. He is snoring uncharacteristically loudly and unevenly. The effort it takes for him to simply breathe propels his chest upward and rattles my senses. I have been sharing a bed with this man for almost twenty-five years. This is not his sound. I sit in the dark and measure the contours of his form under the loose sheet. As usual, both feet poke their way off the edge of the bed. Dennis's toenails need cutting. That has become my job since he isn't strong enough to effectively manage scissors. But today, toenails are low priority. Breathing? That's high priority. I study it. Is he developing aspiration pneumonia as a result of swallowing deficits? That's a common problem when disease process taxes major physical systems (and Dennis has been choking so much lately that I wonder if anything actually goes down the *right* way). You can treat the symptoms— here, the pneumonia—but if their cause remains unchecked, they will reoccur sooner rather than later in most cases. I want to understand what is happening to Dennis, so I can be sure his treatment plan corresponds with our goals. More than anything in the world, I want Dennis to survive this crisis and grow old with me, but only if, as the poet says, "the best is yet to be." I don't want him to suffer like this anymore. I'm aware that these two goals are coming to be mutually exclusive.

Dennis suddenly shudders visibly and drags his forearm over his chest and face, on his way to settling it above his head. A few minutes later, he squints at me through the darkness and says, "I had a nightmare." He asks me to bring him the walker, but then he sobs quietly because he thinks (correctly) that he's now too weak to use it. When Dennis becomes overwhelmed—and that's not often—he lists all his losses like some dwindling inventory at a flea market. "My handwriting is illegible...I can't use a knife...My legs have no muscle mass...My eyes look odd...I can't hit the high notes in 'Danny Boy' anymore..." He rehearses this litany for what seems like much longer than it can really be. Then he begins to weep, face down in that bed. After a time, the flow of tears stops, and Dennis seems to be steeling himself to take a different emotional tack. Suddenly calm, he says, "There is very little I can do. But I can still honor God and love you." His voice cracks and he cries softly, "I just don't know if I can be a blessing anymore." Something in his use of the word "blessing" and the desperation in his voice compel me to help Dennis see the value of his days, specifically of *this* day.

"You can give me a blessing!" I suggest with far more certainty than I feel. "Like in the Old Testament when they invoked the God of Abraham and Isaac and Jacob..." I lay my head down on the bed near his left hand. With my face buried in the bedding and my husband's square hand nestled in my hair, I listen to his voice praying for me. I can't make out the words, but I can sense the blessing. Without moving, I look up into Dennis's face and see a peace that passes understanding. I have read about the peace that only comes from God in the Bible, but I have never witnessed it like this. I know at this moment that there will not be another meltdown. I will also come to know that this is another last: the last time Dennis prays aloud. I treasure the profound sense of that prayerful place where we are able to transcend the harsh realities of impending death.

For us, the world has been reduced to a husband and wife in a hospital room, and I'm savoring every moment with Dennis. After an unknown span of time, I snap out of my reverie and remember the dear friends and family across the country who eagerly await my daily e-mails. I try to give them detailed news as events unfold, but I can't possibly capture the intensity of what is happening.

Perhaps our daughter Juliana's writing some years after Dennis's death tells of the experience most accurately. "I felt like a complete zombie, but I didn't expect physical manifestations. All I could do was stand there and stare at whatever I was supposed to be working on. I've had to call my best friends to come and help me, or they would find me just sitting. And I love them all for understanding even though none of us really knew what was happening. My dad would have known. But I can't call him, and those panic attacks and moments of feeling frozen don't go away just because he did." So go easy on yourself, Other Wife.

When I come back from e-mailing an update, I find Dr. Kara and Jane in the hall outside Dennis's room. Our exchange is brief. We address facets of Dennis's care, specifically the plans for an attempt at palliative sedation—that is, administering enough intravenous medications to give Dennis a drug-induced nap. We've tried everything else, including a full epidural (like they use for childbirth), but nothing has given him one iota of relief. Ideally, Dennis will not only be given respite from his unrelenting pain, but he will also register that pain at some lowered intensity after the structured period of sedation, which is anticipated to be twenty-four hours. I cling to hope but never really think the best-case scenario will transpire. I get the disconcerting sense that nobody else does either. Still, the possibility of a twenty-four-hour nap appeals. All we want is a break in the battle of this war during which such a formidable enemy has had free reign in my husband's body. At this point, that body is both emaciated from lack of intake and a racing metabolism, and swollen from fluid overload. The man who thrust himself into the hospital by sheer will looks like he's been inflated with a bicycle pump and is in danger of a blowout.

In the middle of a practical discussion about the logistics of Dennis's treatment, Dr. Kara freezes. She looks at me intently, and I can tell her agenda has shifted. She opens her mouth, studies me, and then closes it again. Pausing only for a moment, she pulls courage out of the air and blurts, "Do you have supportive relationships?" Thinking she's referring to our vast and wonderful network of friends and family, I assure her there's an army out there. But that's not what she means. Her eyes lock on mine, and she asks if I have a relationship with a therapist, "For when..." Her voice trails back into that deep place in her throat.

I grab at that same reservoir of courage somewhere in the space between us and finish her sentence. "For when Dennis dies?" I ask without breathing.

"Yes. This is going to be the hardest thing you've ever done." She speaks with a frightening but compassionate certainty. I know she means learning how to do life without my best friend, my favorite musician, the father of my complex children, my most insightful political pundit, the president of my fan club, and the man who has prayed for me daily since we met in 1982. I know what Dr. Kara is driving at, but the demands of the day are about as much real life as I can handle, so I try not to think too much about tomorrow and beyond. That's my coping style, and I'm sticking to it. Dr. Kara senses my resolve and leaves me with a quick hug. I wonder what the Other Wife does to stay sane and drift off into an internal conversation with her.

People will accuse you of being in denial if you appear functional at any time during this end-of-life season. Consider it a compliment, Other Wife. Personally, I think denial is underrated. If it works for you, by all means, use it. This time in the hospital is my chance to advocate for Dennis, so he might benefit from all that the US medical system has to offer. There will be days stretching out from here when I can focus on my own loss. Far too many days, I fear. But even now, I know in my heart that the God who gave me

Dennis will sustain me in the days without him. He'll help me, and He'll send people to help me. I know I can't get through this alone. I've already started meeting with a very wise and sympathetic psychiatrist. Just in case nobody in your world has the courage to bring it up like Dr. Kara did for me, let me tell you: you'll benefit immeasurably from the care of a skilled mental health professional when you move toward that place of "Adult You, Part 2." You know how to be a wife. Now you have to learn how to be a widow. Other relationships will also need redefining. You might be a single parent now. You'll have different financial responsibilities. You will often be the third or the fifth, or seated beside the other single person at social events. You'll have to face a deafening silence that your husband's voice once filled. The evenings will get longer and the nights darker. But you will still be you.

Ironically, the faith that sustained Dennis and me through the years, months, and weeks of this illness seem like a strike against us in Dennis's final days. Frank professions of faith make some medical people nervous. Perhaps they fear that people of faith are going to wait for a miracle instead of following professional instructions. Or perhaps they think we are a bit too comfortable with death. When the head of the ethics committee, Dr. Maggie Gallagher, asks me about how the hospital has responded to our faith, I don't hold back. I tell her that our faith appears to be a detriment in our quest for compassionate end-of-life care. I also tell her that if Dennis were to hear me speak those words, he would vehemently disagree or at least kick my vulnerable shins under the table. But I'm beginning to get comfortable speaking for both of us, with a nod to our individual perspectives on life and death.

For his part, lately Dennis speaks and writes constantly about the intimacy suffering has brought to his relationship with God. He shares this perspective in an e-mail to offer a measure of comfort to the countless friends and family searching for a shred of meaning in this cruel time: "For me, it always comes back to Jesus. In the midst of my misery, I strain into him and find solace there. I am comforted by the words of St. Peter in his first epistle where he begins speaking of the refining work of suffering and the product of faith that is 'of greater value than gold.'" But Dennis isn't just preaching. He fills the pages of his private journal with deep reflection on the topic. This is his reality: the Creator who knows Dennis intimately and cares for him beyond any human capacity will sustain him through this pain marring the end of his life. The process of dying and ultimately going to a heaven where his crippled body will no longer confine him doesn't frighten Dennis. He is eager for that day, even though thoughts of leaving our young-adult daughters and me rend his heart.

For my part, as Dennis slips farther away under the increasing burden of his disease, I can see how God has gifted me to be Dennis's companion through this illness and how He will provide for me in its wake. I know that my greatest role in life is as patient advocate in my own husband's room and around his care. In stark contrast to the day Dennis dragged his barely upright body into this hospital, I find myself oddly calm. There are some tears in the dark of the long nights. Yet mostly, I am mindful that the future will hold countless nights where I will long for one more look at Dennis's face, one more touch of his solid, square hands, or one more waft of the scent that has been mine to imbibe for a quarter of a century. I don't want to waste the time we have together. I brace myself against the waves of grief, so I can rest in this quiet place with Dennis for whatever time we have left. I have books and knitting with me but rarely even glance at them. This is my time to soak in as much of Dennis as I possibly can, and I fully delight in that privilege.

Dennis believes that his disease and its progression are no surprise to God. Even if the medical community doesn't understand his illness and has not been able to mitigate its symptoms, God has a purpose in Dennis's suffering. For that reason, the sicker Dennis gets, the more he clings to what he knows to be true of God. He has always prayed and sought truth fervently, but now he's entered into a deeper intimacy with God as a result of this illness. While he still has the strength to speak, Dennis talks about what God is showing him in this dark place. He points to a "calm" and a "sweetness" beyond description and commits over and over again to honor God no matter what trials come.

Trials do seem to cling to Dennis as if to test or taunt. But rather than turning to any other source of hope, Dennis holds ever tighter to his sense that God gives eternal meaning to temporal circumstances. This isn't because Dennis can't continue to trust God as the normal routines of life become increasingly arduous. On the contrary, he's drawing deeply from his faith and the God who informs it in ways he's never experienced before. There are no easy days physically. None. Ever. Without faith, there might well not have been life at all. Certainly there wouldn't be such a rich life that, even as it wanes, remains prayerful and relational at the core.

Again Juliana asked to speak to you, Other Wife.

"One of the last few things I heard from my Dad was the recitation of 'my flesh and my heart might fail, but God is the strength of my heart forever.' Good is still good, and life is still so incredibly beautiful, but even years later, there are many days or parts of days that feel like a cruel joke. Sometimes I wonder if a scan would show a crack in my heart. Maybe the only reason it didn't completely break and kill me was because there was so much love and support keeping all the threads knit together. Maybe it was all the little things that went right on the June day when it all went wrong.

"I remember being terrified of going on in life without my dad to call when I needed something or just to have him there to understand or laugh with me. I really loved being around him, and I was happy when he was with my friends and me. I thought he was so cool. He was always the fun dad. I am still terrified of not having him here. I just can't think of that, or it will become one of those days of sheer torture. You have to force yourself not to think about it all the time, or you won't get out of bed. It's too much for anyone to imagine—so just don't. Half the reason

I found myself starting the day was that the family dog, Yankee, my dad's little shadow, needed to go out. I suggest you get a dog!"

Something remarkable is transpiring, but only Dennis has a clear view of what lies ahead. ("Front row!" he would say if he could.) As his eyes grow dim and his body atrophies, his spirit remains strong. Stronger than ever. Even friends and family who have been skeptical of Dennis's faith in the past are dusting off their Bibles, searching for the source of his incredible strength. Several people recognize Dennis's end-of-life battle in this Bible verse:

> For I am already being poured out like a drink offering, and the time has come for my departure. I have fought the good fight, I have finished the race, I have kept the faith. Now there is in store for me the crown of righteousness, which the Lord, the righteous judge, will award to me on that day—and not only to me but to all who have longed for his appearing. (2 Timothy 4:6–8)

Dennis didn't choose to have this disease quite literally pour him out, but the hope inspired by the promise of a crown at the end of it helped him fight the good fight and keep the faith.

TALKING POINTS FOR MORTALS

1. Are you connected well enough to a spiritual community?
2. How does your faith impact the way that you experience your medical realities?
3. How might your faith be strengthened going forward?

■ ■ ■

CHAPTER 3

DNR

abbr. "do not resuscitate" a medical order that allows the withholding of interventions intended to support pulmonary or cardiac function

Walk the halls of any advanced-care nursing home or hospice, and just about every patient will have dnr posted by his or her bedside. Without a DNR in place, the medical staff is required by law to attempt to resuscitate a dying person, even if it means performing rib-shattering CPR thrusts on a frail elderly woman whose heart has (understandably) stopped. If she survives the ordeal, she will likely live out her days in constant pain or under heavy sedation. Understanding these ramifications, the patient and her family can thoughtfully consider requesting a DNR before she reaches that point. But such decisions are never easy.

Dennis's case was especially complicated. His first DNR came abruptly and, as such, with little opportunity to consider its nuances. About a year prior to his final hospitalization, an inpatient hospice stay was ordered to address a clearly documented pain crisis—that is, pain that was not adequately controlled in a home setting. The plan was to administer high doses of drugs intravenously in various sequences and combinations under the constant watch of clinicians specializing in end-of-life comfort care. So Dennis entered hospice care even though, as far as we knew, death wasn't imminent. This particular hospice center requires a DNR on all patients because it isn't equipped with the technology to monitor and intervene if cardiopulmonary complications arise. Even more, it simply isn't the objective of hospice care to keep someone alive as a goal unto itself. Suffering, not death, is the primary foe. Hospice offers patients individualized care plans that include music therapy, massage, counseling, and chaplain services in addition to medical care. It's all about achieving comfort for those who need it most. And Dennis desperately needed some comfort.

The hospice Dennis entered has a large, bright family room with a television, fully equipped kitchen, comfortable seating, and a computer for family use. They also provide a web service known as CarePages where I could post updates for our family and friends and, hopefully, keep the phones from ringing incessantly. Dennis was allowed to sip wine while the IV was going. For these benefits and the hope of some pain relief, we were willing to sign the consent for a DNR.

Like a prescription for medication or a request for diagnostic testing, "do not resuscitate" is a medical order applied to a patient only by an MD. Anyone can request a DNR, but only a physician can put it in place. When a patient is unable to discuss this order with the MD, a surrogate—a spouse, son, daughter, parent, dear friend, or in some cases a court-appointed guardian—engages with the MD in considering the implications of a DNR order. The red chart label for a DNR is placed prominently at the top of the electronic medical record and on the spine of any paper chart binder. It is arresting, and rightfully so. When a patient's heart stops, the medical staff doesn't have time to fumble around searching for a DNR designation. They will launch into CPR unless they are clearly directed not to.

When a hospital MD pronounces death, three components are noted: absence of breath, absence of heartbeat, and absence of response to painful stimuli. A DNR's implications can be outlined with the same three criteria. It means that there will be no attempt to restart breathing or use of a respirator to facilitate breathing. There will be no CPR or artificial sustaining of a heartbeat. All of this is to increase the likelihood that there will be fewer painful stimuli, less intrusion, and less anxiety surrounding death. A DNR acknowledges the fact that life is ebbing away and that interventions are more likely to prolong the cruel absurdities of the dying process than to extend a life well lived.

This hospice stay was, for us, a dry run of sorts. Dennis was discharged in exactly one month, after which he would return to visit other patients and joke with the nurses about being their favorite "hospice alumnus." But fourteen months later, Dennis's pain had escalated far beyond what he could have imagined at the time of the first hospice stay.

This time he chose to enter one of the city's large research hospitals in his quest for even just a little reprieve from the pain.

Dennis and I had spoken about the DNR option many times in the intervening months between these two hospitalizations, both theoretically, because it is the language of my profession, and personally, because both Dennis and I have complicated medical histories. To be more precise, we each have a personal history of cancer and have lived under what Dennis calls the "C-shaped cloud" for a decade. If surgery and daily radiation don't force discussions of end-of-life care, certainly chemotherapy will. These are heavy conversations for most people, even if you're talking about your eighty-nine-year-old grandpa who's in a coma following a stroke. Our first DNR conversation came when I was in my thirties and our children were still in grade school. At age fifty-two—by no means old in this modem age of medicine—Dennis's consideration of DNR was weighty indeed. As often as I had initiated that discussion and worked to clarify patient and surrogate goals in my professional role as a medical/end-of-life social worker, the questions surrounding a DNR had never before been both so clear and so murky.

So here we are again, back in the hospital, this time jockeying back and forth between the palliative care floor where Dennis has been admitted and the ICU where even higher doses of narcotics are to be administered. Dennis is very, very sick and feeling extraordinarily vulnerable. He's quite literally engaging in his own life-and-death discussion while lying on a table in a hospital gown surrounded by pensive, top-notch professionals. What a far cry from the years he spent at the fronts of boardrooms dressed in well-tailored business suits closing those proverbial million-dollar deals. After a thorough and prayerful consideration of his options, Dennis confirms his wish to proceed as a DNR patient for the remainder of the treatments being recommended for him by the palliative care team. That's what we're here for: full palliative sedation under the vigilance of the hospital's ICU staff. Dennis hasn't wavered in the thinking he shared with me while he was dressed and sitting at home, but now he is being forced to defend his stance to medical professionals on their turf.

> *I keep thinking of you, my dear Other Wife. This is such a difficult discussion to have even in the privacy of your own home. In the hospital, they expect you to have it with an audience. And that audience is not typically eager to use a DNR for anyone they deem reasonably healthy and young. (In my experience, reasonably healthy means breathing, and young is under eighty-five.) So you, like so many of the hospital staff, must be wondering why I stand in support of enforcing a DNR status in my still-conversant fifty-two-year-old husband. You have good reason to ask, and I will answer honestly. Dennis's suffering is so thoroughly awful that two months before he entered the hospital he penned this in his journal:*
>
> *"My earliest flirtations with suicide began over a year ago and shocked me. I had moved into a realm that was utterly foreign to anything I had ever*

experienced. I lost control of so much and permanently lost my ability to run, play basketball, play tennis, ski, go for long walks with Susan, hike, swim, or sit and watch movies, concerts, lyric opera, ballet...And then, in the prime of my career, I lost that too (and the dreams of making a financial impact through giving). And piled on top of [these] losses is a twenty-four-hour battle with unremitting pain. My [disease] promises to continue to introduce new losses and new sources of pain without any relief from the current situation. My right hand continues to weaken. It is very hard to write this. Blindness lurks as a real possibility. My voice quality is rapidly deteriorating..." (04.13.08)

This is just a glimpse of Dennis's reality as he experienced it. I wonder what you're dealing with right now, Other Wife. As surely as your circumstances differ from ours, your choices and decisions will vary across the spectrum. I don't know how to advise you, but I long to reach out to you and offer an understanding ear.

Time and time again, Dennis told me that he would never take his own life because, quite simply, his faith in a sovereign God precludes it. There was also the matter of his commitment to our daughters and me. No, Dennis wouldn't do more than flirt with taking his own life, but his resolve against suicide is a matter of conviction not desire. Dennis's strong convictions always win the internal tug-of-war between life and death, but his desire for an escape from this agony haunts him day and night.

Dennis isn't choosing death by opting to enter the ICU with a DNR in place. He just doesn't want to end up receiving treatment that would leave him trapped in a dying body, unable to even writhe away from his unrelenting pain. Given his choice, he'd like to live to be an old man. He wants to celebrate milestones with his children and welcome his as-yet-unborn grandchildren. But this complex pain syndrome, the ravages of which those of us watching can only barely imagine, has robbed him of the ability to enjoy any facet of life. There really are fates worse than death.

Dealing with a DNR in the intensive care unit of a large, urban research hospital is a whole different experience from the relatively charmed hospice stay Dennis had fourteen long months ago. Today as Dennis leaves the hospital's palliative care floor and is wheeled on a gurney into the underground passages that snake between buildings, the framed floral prints do nothing to soften the oversized squares of grazed linoleum and hospital-neutral paint. Periodically, the man pushing the gurney uses his ID to command a heavy pair of metal doors to divide. But they rarely open in unison, so I dash ahead of the gurney to hold them apart. My back presses against their weight as I hug a gigantic Ziploc bag labeled personal belongings in my arms. I'm struck by the pride I feel in doing *something* for Dennis. Anything. Dennis doesn't appear to notice much about the underground tour. He doesn't inquire about his favorite T-shirts and slippers. Even more unusual, he doesn't ask the man steering the gurney anything about himself. My husband's world has diminished to the point where all he notices is the trajectory of the little mattress on wheels.

Our arrival at the ICU is met with much scurrying. The constant, deliberate movement of serious-faced professionals makes me feel like we accidentally wandered into a NASA space center in the midst of a major launch. I know from working as a social worker in the ICU that the urgency of this place typically overwhelms patients and their families.

I would hate for you, dear Other Wife, to be unduly anxious. You have enough on your mind, and I know your heart is heavy. Don't let the ICU's high-tech sights and sounds distract you from what you're here to do. The staff on these units is crackerjack good. Because they're trained to deal with crises, their approach can seem mechanical and hurried. But they don't mean to distance themselves from you. If you need them to explain something, you should feel free to ask. Most of them are terrific educators with a passion for what they do. They worry sometimes that family will get in the way, but that's just because they're focused on giving the very best care possible. I've found that if I'm quick to step back from the bed when they approach, and ask for permission before doing seemingly small things like changing the elevation of the head of the bed or repositioning an arm, they appear less irritated by my presence.

This day, Dennis and I are met by three energetic young nurses who immediately set to work establishing scientific data on what is happening to Dennis's body. They press cardiac leads onto his atrophied chest and deftly tuck a blood pressure cuff around what was once an impressive enough bicep. Then they snap what looks like a white plastic clothespin onto his right index finger, which from then on gives off a Rudolph-like red glow as it measures Dennis's blood-oxygen level. It doesn't seem to matter that this renders the hand pretty much useless. What is he going to do with it anyway? While all of these machines allow Dennis's vital signs to be closely observed, I have a sinking sense that he—my real Dennis—is becoming increasingly less visible in the ways that matter to me: the warmth of his smile, the mischief in his eyes, and the assurance of his gentle but firm touch.

Just as the senior resident who introduced herself earlier in the day arrives on the scene, Dr. Mark Bjorn, the pulmonologist overseeing Dennis's care on the ICU, comes to "verify that we're all on the same page." Discussions that start this way end well only if they're not needed in the first place. I doubt this will be an exception. Members of the ICU team have a considerable stake in coercing Dennis to begin his treatment at what is referred to as a "full code," meaning that every attempt will be made to sustain life should Dennis's current crisis become life threatening. For example, if Dennis's breathing becomes compromised while he's under sedation, they want the go-ahead to insert a tube down his throat to enable a breathing machine to mechanically inflate his lungs. If the ICU has a mission statement, it could be summed up as, "Keep the patient breathing." If that needs to be done by a machine, then so be it. After patients are stable on machines, they are transferred to a facility specializing in managing the care of people who live with tubes in their throats. As you can imagine, intubation makes speaking very arduous, if at all possible, and eating, moving, and participating in life in any active way virtually impossible. I'm not a fan of such a lifestyle in most cases, and in Dennis's case, the complications would be profound because his central nervous system pain syndrome makes staying in any one position for any length of time excruciatingly painful.

> *How would your beloved want his care to proceed, Other Wife? Talk with him about these choices in advance, if you can. But if you can't, get some good counsel. Ask lots of questions. It's one of the most significant decisions you'll make. Don't go it alone.*

Both the palliative team and the ICU team interfacing in Dennis's transfer ask repeatedly during the course of this afternoon how Dennis would like to handle the code status. He's fairly clear about his wishes, initially. When the MDs probe a bit more and ask about scenarios in which intubation might be needed as a stop-gap measure to guard his life should he not be able to "protect his airways," his face radiates fear. He looks to me to get his bearings. When the professionals leave the room, he and I review what we understand to be happening medically in his unique case. I assure Dennis that when he is sedated and unable to articulate his wishes, I will be in that room with him constantly, and I will advocate for his best interest with everything in me.

Dr. Kara from the palliative floor has given me her personal cell phone number, specifically stating that she sleeps with that phone by her bed. She tells me that I should feel free to call if I have any concerns through the night. I think to myself, "This woman, who clearly puts in twelve-plus hour days at the hospital, deserves a night's rest." As if she can read my mind, she counters, "If it weren't okay to call, I wouldn't have given you the number," as she heads down the hall. As it turns out, I won't need to wake her tonight. I need her help before she even leaves the hospital.

I have followed Dennis's gurney from the palliative floor to the ICU, where hospital protocol requires him to remain for the administration of a short-acting anesthetic called Versed. This is deemed necessary because, aside from putting people in a twilight sleep with no memory of events transpired, the drug suppresses respiration. In the event that a patient can't protect his own airways with reflexive coughing, repositioning, or swallowing, intubation with a respirator is readily available. Perhaps even more important, the staff on an ICU is especially skilled in these procedures. This life-saving technology is their passion and the reason many of them choose to work these units. Dennis isn't just a patient to these people. He's a professional challenge.

I make the mistake of leaving Dennis's room for two minutes in order to use the bathroom an hour after we arrive on the ICU. When I return, Dennis looks shaken. "The pulmonologist was here. He says I'm 'tying his hands' by wanting the sedation but not authorizing the use of a breathing tube. I told him I needed to wait until you were here to decide what to do."

My husband and I revisit how terribly ill he is and how difficult life has become for him. We talk about his prognosis. We both know that he will continue to decline at some unknown but likely precipitous rate until his body can no longer sustain life. We talk about the ultimate goals of his medical care: to live whatever is left of life with as little pain as possible. He is clear on all of these things, but the pulmonologist's anxiety about the DNR causes my already distressed husband to second-guess his own wishes. MDs have tremendous influence on the emotional states of their patients. I often wonder how many MDs understand the position of power they hold vis-à-vis their patients.

Part of Dennis's response to the doctor's questioning is raw fear at the realities he faces medically. But it also stems from the fact that he has a competitive streak but no personal tolerance for discord. My husband is a peacemaker who, by temperament, isn't equipped to fix a stake in the ground for his own benefit. It seems to matter so much to this pulmonologist and his staff that Dennis not proceed with a DNR in place that Dennis might be swayed to agree to be a full code. But I have seen too much of what happens to terminally ill patients who are intubated. These visions frighten me more than any dispute we may have with the MD in charge of the ICU.

A have an idea that might help Dennis weigh his options. "I'll walk around this ICU and tell you how many beds there are and how many have patients who are breathing on their own, okay?" I do a quick tour. Of twenty-six beds, I count on one hand those without ventilators in use. Indeed, the goal of care on this unit is to get people discharged from its cubicles breathing, more often than not with assistance. The staff on an ICU is an A-team committed to this goal. But their short-term agenda is often diametrically opposed to the goals of palliative care. The philosophy behind palliative medicine hinges on a "less is more" approach in terms of technology, promoting an interdisciplinary model of care instead. I always think of palliative care as the modem-day equivalent of an old-fashioned, small-town community where we're all in this together. But I feel torn in encouraging Dennis to remain a DNR because I know we're asking the ICU staff to step outside of their comfort zone and administer a very different sort of care than they've been trained to offer. This work is their passion, after all.

It's becoming clear that a palliative patient should never be transferred to the ICU. As it turns out, after Dennis's experience, the hospital will change its protocol so palliative patients with DNR designations will receive their treatments on the palliative floors. But that fight is as yet to be won this day on the ICU.

The pulmonologist reappears. Dennis tells him he does indeed want to remain both a DNR and a DNI (Do Not Intubate). Some patients are willing to allow a breathing tube but not the often violent intervention of the chest compressions and electrical shock used to restart a heart, should it for any reason stop beating. The pulmonologist seems frustrated and flustered. He repeats for my benefit what he said to Dennis earlier: "Because of the high rate of sedation, Dennis might not be able to protect his airway. If he were to choke on secretions, he might not be able to breathe. Without the freedom to intubate

Dennis, this treatment could be life threatening." He shifts from one foot to another waiting for a response from us, his eyes darting around the room. I know that Dennis has every legal right to elect a DNR/DNI. But this MD clearly believes this is either wrong in general or a wrong use of the ICU. On the latter point I agree with him, but we are at an impasse.

I need Dr. Kara. I page her. When she responds, I tell her we're having trouble regarding the DNR. She arrives so quickly I wonder if Scotty has beamed her to the ICU *Star Trek* style. The staccato click of her heels announces her arrival, indicating by its sharp cadence that she is on a mission. I instantly draw strength from her energy and resolve. Dr. Kara spends a couple of minutes verifying what is happening and then disappears into the center of the unit to find the pulmonologist. I hear them discussing the DNR issue outside Dennis's temporary house of glass. Dr. Bjorn sounds irritated. Dr. Kara sounds resolute. Unthwarted by my usual no-eavesdropping policy, I strain to make out their words. I miss most of the details, but I do catch a pejorative reference to MDs who don't understand how quickly things can go bad in an ICU. And I catch part of the rebuttal judiciously mixed with some deference.

When the two MDs enter Dennis's room, Dr. Kara begins by addressing me. "I think it'll be best if we all have the same conversation." I'm unwavering in my commitment to keep the DNR, but Dennis is exhausted and at times appears confused. He asks questions to which I'm sure he already knows the answers and looks to me for reassurance at every turn.

"If it's just for an hour or two maybe that would be okay?" he asks me with fear in his eyes.

"I'll be right here the whole time. If that's what the situation calls for, we can just go with it," I assure him. Dennis's eyes remain fixed on me, and the fear begins to fade from their piercing blueness. Before anyone can exhale, Dr. Bjorn says he would prefer to hear from Dennis himself what his desire is before we proceed. Fair enough. This stance is not only morally sound, it complies with the law. Patients must make their own health care decisions as long as they are competent to do so. Eventually, we get clarity and the DNR/DNI stands. I thank Dr. Kara for coming to the rescue. I assume that I will have no further need for her that night, but knowing where I am, I check to be sure I haven't misplaced her cell phone number—twice—before she leaves.

Even as I marshal all my intellectual conviction to convince the Smart People (as I respectfully dub the hospital staff) that Dennis and I really do know what we're doing, my own emotions turn on me. Doubts creep in. What if indeed this end-of-life crisis is a result of medical intervention, as a small contingent of professionals is asserting? What if it can indeed be reversed? What if Dennis is not merely flummoxed and would actually like to accept a full-code status? What would my daughters think if they knew of this scenario? If I bring my Dream Man home on hospice, how will I handle the administration of potentially lethal medication? Under all of this pressure, I ask myself, "Am I brave enough to advocate for this man in this situation and live with the consequences, whatever they may be?"

And I wonder if you, dear Other Wife, also face some of these larger-than-life questions. I pray God will grant us the courage to do what is best for the ones who need our help, now.

The stream of MDs, APNs, RNs, and seemingly every other clinical staff member in this large teaching hospital traipsing through the ICU awakens me (and my existential questions) intermittently throughout the night. They're all wide awake and curious about Dennis's unusual case, which has created a buzz about "the patient on the ICU with a DNR." They stop by "just to check," "wanting to verify," "clarifying that," "wondering if you understand the implications." All I can tell them is, indeed, the DNR is firmly in place. Knowing that Dennis's status contradicts the ICU's mission to protect airways, I make every effort to be gracious with these emissaries, even as stifled screams of angst and rage lay dormant in my own perfectly functional lungs.

Lying on a sheet on the floor of the ICU, I discover that the noises characteristic of this place echo louder in the night when fewer—if not few—bodies move around to absorb them. Mechanistic hums and whirs are punctuated with irregular alarms and insistent beeps. Peaks and valleys in Dennis's body function variously measured by modern technology trigger an occasional alarm. Other sounds simply announce the passage of hospital ritual: the medication bag is empty, a bolus of medication is not yet allowed, or perhaps IV lines need adjustment. The machine usually spells out in an arresting, red techno-font that "lines are occluded—patient side," as if even under full sedation and restraints, Dennis is to blame. In truth, it's more often his wife whose arm has settled on a line nestled in bedding or whose leaning in to kiss his cheek has annoyed the system. I'm sure I'm annoying the staff here even more.

I try not to take it personally when the staff treats me like an unwelcome guest in their ICU. You shouldn't either, Other Wife. You know you're right where you need to be.

Winding down her day well into the night as Dennis begins his twenty-sixth hour in the ICU, Dr. Kara's heels announce her approach once again. This time they offer a less urgent and more comforting clip-tick. Dr. Kara seems more interested in how Dennis appears to be doing than in what some discrete or objective measurements of technology reveal. I don't even know if she looks at the monitors. Her focus is my husband. She speaks directly to him, but he shows no sign of comprehension. He is, after all, heavily sedated. That fact notwithstanding, he moans quietly and shakes his furrowed head as if trying to clear cobwebs. His wrists and ankles are, at this point, in soft restraints. Dr. Kara gives me the go-ahead to remove them. Doing so makes me feel that Dennis is somehow doing better, even though I know this really didn't change anything. It just means I have a greater responsibility to watch him even more closely. Watching Dennis is my only commitment as these hours collect into days.

I lean toward Dr. Kara and, in a groggy whisper, ask her not to disturb Dennis. At this point my only reflex is to protect Dennis, but I realize now how silly my request was. He gives no indication of being aware of anything going on around him. But the pain within his body still shows itself in his grimacing face, even at a dosage 225 times beyond that which usually renders a patient unaware of pain.

I'm not exaggerating, Other Wife! They've really hit him with a drug combination 225 times more potent than the norm. What next?

"The pulmonologist says we've hit the maximum dose of Versed he'll authorize," I report to Dr. Kara.

After a comment about the rate of infusion, she shrugs and agrees. "I don't think it should go higher either."

So we review the course of events. As she continues to rehash the harrowing details of the previous day, I find myself becoming increasingly light-headed and nauseated. I look down at Dr. Kara's shoes, fairly sure I'm about to empty the contents of my stomach on them. Thankfully, her pager interrupts. As she excuses herself, I sit on the floor leaning over the pullout commode wondering why I suddenly feel so ill. Apparently, discussing the rate and means by which your husband is dying will do that to a person who hasn't eaten or slept much for quite some time. When Dr. Kara returns I have steeled myself against whatever might happen next, but I'm newly aware that my own health is becoming a factor alongside Dennis's. I resolve to be more responsible with the limited resource known as me.

How are you feeling, Other Wife? Are you getting any rest? Are you eating anything remotely nutritious? Just as flight attendants always instruct travelers to "place the oxygen mask on yourself before you assist the person next to you," try to take care of yourself in this extremely stressful time. You won't be any help to your husband if you faint from hunger or exhaustion.

The worst of my little spell is over by the time Dr. Kara returns. "We'll keep Dennis here overnight for monitoring and then transfer him back to the floor in the morning. I have a bed reserved for him," she offers.

"Since he's not getting any more Versed, does protocol allow him to go back to the floor now rather than waiting till morning?" I ask gently, trying not to sound as desperate as I feel. Dr. Kara hears my plea, and soon Dennis is prepped and heading back through the subterranean maze to the palliative floor.

Dr. Bjorn, who railed against the DNR the day before, examines Dennis one last time before we leave the ICU—*his* ICU. I recall how he washed his hands meticulously when he entered Dennis's room for the first time as I watch him approach the sink once more. While plunging his hands into the running water, he looks over his left shoulder. His eyes scan Dennis's sinking form on their way to meet mine. "He's very fortunate to have you as his wife," he states as a matter of fact. Before I can grasp this olive branch, he dries his hands and walks out the door as if cleansed from the whole ordeal.

Within the hour, Dennis and I return to a room on the palliative floor with a recliner and a window and food service and familiar RNs who greet us warmly. In contrast to the ICU, this is a staggeringly wonderful place. It feels like a safe place for Dennis, which makes it a haven for me as well. I flop into the recliner with a sigh of relief and a smile. That my joy should be so palpable in the middle of what I am becoming more and more sure are my Dennis's last days surprises me, but I'll take any comfort I can get right now. I know the challenges awaiting us will be no less arduous and the truths we must face no less harsh here on the palliative floor. Still, the environment—by protocol—is the right place for us. Sinking deeper into my recliner, I realize I have gone from nauseated to giddy in less than an hour.

TALKING POINTS FOR MORTALS

1. Do you understand this term - DNR - and how it might apply to your medical realities, either now or in the future as disease progresses?

2. Do your loved ones and medical team know how much technology you want used at the end of your life?

■ ■ ■

CHAPTER 4

Protocol

[proh-tuh-kawl] n. detailed clinical guidelines designed to increase quality of care and decrease risk

As I send daily updates to the multitudes of friends and family glued to our CarePage blog, I must weigh how much to communicate with them. I covet their prayers and am clear that, although I've asked them to refrain from visiting Dennis (and me) during this hospitalization, knowing we have a personal army supporting us in every conceivable way precludes any sense of my being a lone warrior. Omitting most of the harrowing details of the ICU fiasco, I decide to take a forward-looking approach in this morning's report:

> Okay, so the ICU stint ended last night when Dennis did not appear to be benefiting from CRAZY doses of sedation. (He did stop the writhing in the bed but not the frowning and groaning

that he does unconsciously when he thinks that you and I are not looking and worrying.) We are now on the palliative floor again, where Dennis is slowly becoming more alert. Since no one has ever seen the level of sedation he was given (and no, we are not in a small rural hospital in Tibet!) no one knows how long this will take. Tomorrow he will likely start one of two IV trials with the ongoing goal of getting him comfortable. Dennis has a phenomenal medical team, and we are confident that, where there is anything that can be done to help him, it will be.

With the drug dosages far exceeding the human norm, I have to agree with the pulmonologist that Dennis has "failed" yet another attempt at pain management. Even with a highly unusual abandonment of protocol, the ICU was unable to deliver the relief we had hoped for. As the pain marches on unthwarted, some of the nation's best medical minds go back to the drawing board while Dennis and I hunker down and gird ourselves for whatever the future holds.

Yesterday, an anesthesiologist snaked a sterile line into Dennis's spine for another trial, similar to the type of epidural procedure that gives women pain-free childbirth. If this mode of medication administration could offer Dennis some relief, a permanent version with a refillable, battery-driven pump would be inserted beneath his skin. After learning the intricate details of how the permanent pump would be maintained over the coming months, I was asked to sign informed-consent papers. "Informed consent" is one of my favorite oxymorons in medical care. Your signature on this form indicates that you know what you're getting into when you accept a given treatment. But you're never fully informed because that would mean being able to predict future outcomes. It just isn't possible. So I signed my name on Dennis's chart and prayed this method would be the silver bullet we've been searching for.

> *I would bet that most MDs would really like to tell you everything you need to know to make an informed decision, Other Wife. But they often just don't know. There's rarely enough time to communicate even what they do know. It's also very difficult for professionals in a field as complex as medicine to remember that what's common knowledge to them is completely foreign to a layperson. So keep asking questions until you get an answer you can digest.*

Within a couple of hours of beginning this epidural infusion, there was no indication that the medication was impacting Dennis's pain. He did, however, begin to sweat profusely as a hive-like rash spread rapidly across his chest, shoulders, and neck. The drug infusion was stopped on the assumption that this was an allergic reaction. Nonetheless, today, the same anesthesiologist who initiated the trial arrives in Dennis's room with plans to implant the permanent version. Obviously, I'm not an expert in such things, but I'm not inclined to support an invasive procedure to make permanent something that wasn't helpful temporarily. I ask if the existing line might be removed and this course of treatment discontinued. The MD obliges.

> *If a procedure appears counterintuitive, Other Wife, don't hesitate to voice your opinion. Signing an informed consent form doesn't mean you can't speak up.*

After the anesthesiologist leaves, I notice a new drug bag with an unfamiliar, multisyllabic name hanging on Dennis's IV pole. I ask the nurse about it the next time she comes into the room.

"What is that drug?"

"An antibiotic."

"Why is Dennis on an antibiotic?"

"Because of his fever."

"But we're doing only Tylenol for comfort, no antibiotics."

Unable to respond to my challenge, the nurse goes looking for the MD who prescribed the antibiotic. When she returns, I'm told that "an order was put in to remind us to ask you how you want to treat fevers." Good thing I'm not afraid to ask questions. This is a critical protocol divide. If a patient is expected to recover from whatever else is going on, antibiotics are a wonderful tool in stemming infections. But if patients are being treated for comfort at the end of life, these same antibiotics are often not worth the potential side effects. We opted against the use of antibiotics, but this information wasn't charted. Without proper documentation of personal choice, hospitals make decisions based on protocol.

I wonder if you, Other Wife, understand all of this hospital talk of "protocols." The word comes up constantly in a tone bordering on reverence, as if protocol is somehow sacred. But protocol is really just a fancy word for "what we do here."

We all follow protocol to some degree in our daily lives. It may be the routine we follow getting everyone out the door in the morning. It may be the winding down routine at night. Or it might be a protocol for doing laundry or preparing a presentation at work. In a medical setting, protocol has far-reaching implications. Protocols exist to implement best-practice guidelines across the spectrum of hospital scenarios. They are intended to guard the quality of care and the perception of patient service through both straightforward experiences and those that deviate from every conceivable norm. When events are progressing smoothly, staff might well forget that protocols are encoded for everything from how to reduce infection rates in the operating room to how to handle a hysterical family member receiving frightening news. But when there is an untoward event, or a series thereof, everyone goes scurrying to the hard drives to download policies and protocols. Where current protocols have been violated, there will be extra scrutiny. Where they have been followed but there are still great concerns about outcomes, protocol will be analyzed to see if language, assumptions, applications might be modified. This is best practice. This is personal medical care in the middle of a large institution within a sprawling industry. It's also litigation avoidance.

Three days into our hospital stay, Dennis's care has already challenged hospital protocol in a number of ways. Although I try to go by the rules in most circumstances, I learn to look beyond them during this extraordinary time. Hospital protocol is powerful but not immovable.

Sometimes you have to jump through hoops if you want to challenge the status quo, Other Wife. Just do it, and be ready to pick yourself up and try again if the hoops seem to move while you're in mid-air. There are other times—sweet times—when the hospital staff holds the hoop steady and helps you get through it. Savor those times, and know that your input can shape protocol. Don't be shy about advocating for the one you love dearly, even if it means coloring outside the lines a bit.

This day I am surprised by one of those sweet instances of protocol bending. The staff on the palliative floor encourages me to eat the food that is intended for Dennis. The room comes with food for the patient—part of the spa package. In this particular hospital, the food is outstanding. (No joke!) For the first day or so when Dennis is alert enough to select what he would like to eat, I call his order to the kitchen, and within an hour it arrives: strict protocol at work. For myself, I buy fruit and sandwiches and an occasional something chocolate from the hospital cafe. Soon, however, Dennis is not alert enough to choose menu items or to feed himself when the food arrives. I order soft foods that will be easily digested: Jell-O, creamed soups, macaroni and cheese, none of which I care to eat. After the first day, he subsists only on Jell-O, which stains his thrush-afflicted mouth an orange hue that reminds me of a preschooler after a Halloween party. Then he stops eating even the Jell-O. I am, however, still in need of three meals a day. Both Jennifer Clark, the wonderful RN serendipitously assigned to Dennis during the majority of his stay, and Dr. Kara encourage a variant on protocol: "Meals come with the room rate. Dennis cannot eat. You can eat. Order what *you* will enjoy, given that Dennis is not likely to be eating." I am reminded not to mention this to the kitchen staff when I order, but I doubt I'm fooling anyone. When they bring the tray, the food service staff invariably asks where I would like it placed. I guess they sense that the over bed table is not the right spot. At the end of each meal, the food service person reappears, observes my ever-more-faded husband mouth-breathing and moaning in that bed, and then looks back at the empty tray and me. Collusion. Here, best practice means breaking protocol

Other times the staff seems to taunt you with the elusive hoop and make you shoot for it blindfolded. Like back in the ICU. There Dennis was officially listed NPO (Latin acronym for "nothing by mouth"). There was one small metal chair in the room (think overflow at a school board meeting). There was a pullout commode near the bedside that is rarely used by patients but rather serves as a receptacle where RNs empty catheter bags. The visiting hours posted on the door are 9:00 a.m. to 9:00 p.m., but as you already know, I had no intention of leaving Dennis for even a minute. My one trip down the hall earlier had left him vulnerable to the possibility of intubation. As the night progressed and merged into a new day, I was more committed than ever to my sentry post. Equipped with an apple and a banana and the pullout commode, I figured I could stay in that room for a twenty-four- or thirty-six-hour run without seriously jeopardizing my own health. But there was the matter of sleep. I asked the RN for a sheet to put on the floor, assuring her that I would stay out of her way. She didn't look too thrilled, but she did comply with my request. I thought maybe I was winning her over when she brought me a pair of light blue tube socks too. For my part, I did as promised and placed my sheet a reasonable distance from the bed.

I try to connect with each person attending to Dennis. How committed will they be to him if I'm not respectful—even warm—toward them? In a hospital in general, and around critical care especially, the relationship between the medical team and the patient team is very important. I certainly don't think of Dennis as just one more patient, and I don't want those caring for him to either. That said, this can be easier said than done, particularly in the ICU. Even after the eventful bedside conference regarding the DNR at the beginning of our stay, the fact remained that what was being done—aggressive use of medication for palliation without intubation—*was* permitted by protocol. It's just that this particular protocol was rarely practiced. As such, the ICU staff was very uncomfortable with it. I can only imagine what was being said at the nurses' station out of earshot. Residents and interns and APNs and RNs trolled the ICU all night long, and as I already pointed out, not one seemed to miss a stop at Dennis's bedside. I'll never know if it was disbelief, curiosity, or conscientious objection that fueled the visits. But as the medication doses were ratcheted up according to plan, I was left to fend off the well-meaning intrusions of the night shift:

"I just want to verify that Mr. Sheehan is a DNR and that you don't want him intubated..."

"You know that we have never seen Versed given in such high doses, and so I want to be sure that you understand..."

"It does not appear that he is comfortable yet, but I'm not sure how much more medication we can give him..."

"We need to put restraints on him. He's hallucinating..."

"Would you be willing to allow Dennis to be intubated if his respiration rate drops...?"

"Do you understand that your husband might not be able to protect his airways as we increase the medication...?"

With each of these people, I did my best to be respectful and sympathetic to their perspective. Remember the ICU's agenda—to keep people breathing, get them stabilized, and send them off the unit alive. Conversely, remember the goals Dennis and I had established with the palliative team: to attempt full sedation of a terminally ill man. Even in the midst of this attempt, I understood the dilemma and tried to be patient with the relentless inquisition.

In the midst of this darkness, I find myself thinking about you, Other Wife. Would you have been able to convince the RN to let you sleep on the floor after visiting hours had ended? Do you even know that you can do that? And I wonder how you would handle the well-intentioned harangue launched by every professional within range of the ICU. I'm sure you'd be exhausted, which in itself wears down your mental strength. Then there's that feeling that you're the only person in the world—or at least the only awake person—who thinks that the decisions previously made under less duress are still the best course of action. In my frustration, I pray that you will have peace through the night. I wonder over and over how I can warn you of what you might face. And then I imagine that maybe I would have the privilege of writing to you when my own drama subsides.

The ICU dilemma existed not because the professionals were uncaring, but simply because their agenda was so different from Dennis's and mine. I wanted to scream at these people: "You don't know how hard this is for me to do! I want more than anything in the world for my husband to be well and to come home with me and share life again. But that is not possible, and so I want you to help me honor him by doing everything possible to allow him some measure of comfort as his life winds itself down." I also wanted desperately to hide from the professionals what I was really feeling: "It's really scary to watch you restrain Dennis. Is it really necessary? I care more than you will ever know, and as much as my request goes against your protocols, your actions sure go against mine."

I wished I could tell them that sometimes if you really, really love someone, you have to pretend to be braver than you are on the inside just to do what needs to be done on the outside. And being asked all night long if I was sure about what I was doing? I thought at the time that there was likely a legal case for harassment, but I am not a litigious person. Litigation can only yield money and likely bitterness. There is no legal settlement that will give us back the people we love.

I have to remind myself repeatedly that the people involved in my husband's care are not my enemies. And for Dennis's sake, I find ways to partner with them. Well, most of them. The lady at the desk on the sixteenth floor takes her job very seriously. Emanating a faint aroma of talcum powder and coffee, she somehow appears to be both very busy and totally bored. She does not smile at me, even when I dig to the depths of my soul to find a smile for her. Her eyes narrow as she measures each person passing her. She patrols the elevators. No one without staff identification or a temporary visitor's pass can sneak past her onto the floor. That is the rule. I understand the rule and am happy to comply. But remember that I am sleeping in Dennis's room. Each morning after I shower, I stride past her to get a large chai latte—nonfat, no water, 190 degrees, please. The visitor's pass I wear boldly on my sweater has always expired a few hours earlier at midnight. The first morning I cheerfully explain my situation and assure my adjudicator that I will get my latte and a new badge before coming back to the floor. She is not happy with the plan. When I return with my updated tag a few minutes later, she is not any happier.

On subsequent mornings we reenact this same skit. It seems to me that anyone whose spouse is dying should be treated with some deference. But I guess hospitals are full of soon-to-be widows, so I should not expect any special treatment. Each day I become progressively wearier as my days and nights jumble together and pull apart. I am getting edgy. Walking through the early morning quiet of the hospital halls, I decide to say something to this woman. I start with my customary "good morning" and brace to follow with something short but poignant. And then? Well, she shocks my socks off with a broad smile and a bright "good morning!" Maybe she sensed my new approach. Maybe her sister apologized or one of her kids got a good report card or her husband remembered their anniversary or…whatever. Certainly I am not the only one in the world with challenges, and it is likely good for me to be reminded of that fact.

That experience, Other Wife, reminded me yet again that hospital people are really just people. They will have good days and bad days, and you will be stuck with whatever they bring to work. It is so easy when you are exhausted and frightened and grieving to think that hospital people should understand. Perhaps, but this is life on earth, and they will not always be able to meet us where we would like them to minister one form of grace or another. I play a little game in my head sometimes that might help you. When other people discourage me, I watch for the rudest, most callous, absurd behavior. Then I challenge myself to see if it will be trumped. It distracts me. Sometimes it amuses me. On some occasions it helps me see past myself.

There will always be vagaries in a system as complex as the people who comprise that system. Yet there do seem to be some relatively easy fixes that would facilitate dying well as a matter of protocol. After palliative care is elected by the patient system, any hospitalizations should—must—allow for a bed in a palliative unit. The twenty-six hours that Dennis spent in the ICU were hellacious. The pulmonologist's impassioned assertion that the DNR-DNI Dennis had in place was "tying his hands" proves the incompatibility of these two branches of medicine when placed under pressure. Residents, interns, students, and RNs paraded through Dennis's curtained room as if it were some sort of circus freak show. I assume that most of them had read the chart. I suspect there were many conversations between these professionals about this extraordinary case being lived out in the room on the corner of the unit. They could not get their clinical commitment to "protect an airway" out of their assessment and care of this palliative patient. To be asked to stand firm in the wake of such a tsunami of tension is not fair to patients and their loved ones. Nor is it fair to the ICU team. Protocol was changed, and I rejoice thinking of other families who will never know that particular nightmare.

It was at the end of twenty-six hours on the ICU that I experienced my only physical frailty of those ten days. I had elected not to eat because I knew better than to leave Dennis even for a minute, as his respiratory status was increasingly compromised. But it was not the lack of food that broke me. It was the tension of guarding my husband

and of wanting to be both gracious and clear with staff members whom I believe were well-intentioned...but out of line. I was so nauseated that I rested my head on the side of a porcelain basin, fully expecting to vomit. I did not.

TALKING POINTS FOR MORTALS

1. What routines are important to you in spite of your illness?
2. How have you seen your treatment team to be bound or contracted by established practices?
3. Do you feel able to advocate for an exception or a change in these practices?

∎ ∎ ∎

CHAPTER 5

POA

abbr. "power of attorney" 1. a legal document naming a proxy in the event that direct patient communication is impossible;
2. the person appointed to make medical decisions on behalf of an incapacitated patient

As a medical social worker, I often wish that I could offer the bleary-eyed, strung-out families I work with some medication. They typically look more uncomfortable than the dear one over whose bed they hover. Most hospitals don't even proffer a cup of coffee. You've likely noticed that already, Other Wife. How often have you seen a blanket being adjusted on your husband and thought "I could use one of those; this place is freezing"? And, more often than not, the place is freezing. Hospitals in general and ICUs and ORs in particular are kept cool in order to mitigate the spread of infections. This should be reassuring, I guess, but that doesn't keep your teeth from chattering.

As you sit beside your hospitalized beloved bundled in your coat, you may be wondering about this POA form to which the staff keeps referring. Apparently, you have been named your husband's power of attorney for health care. Everyone acts like you should know what this means, but I know that you might not be sure. You may have guessed the POA is like a will, which is not entirely inaccurate, except that this form has nothing to do with money. I think it is the word "attorney" that confuses people. Oddly enough, this happens to be one of only a few legal documents that can be prepared without an attorney at all. By law, it is offered to everyone who is admitted to a hospital as a free service, but it is not required to receive care. Usually a social worker helps you fill it out. (Dennis and I completed these forms at home because I am one of those social workers.) Essentially, the health care POA is a legal document in which you indicate two things: 1. How you would like end-of-life care handled in terms of the use of technology, and 2. Who you would like to speak on your behalf in the event that you are unable to speak for yourself.

Some people call it a "living will," a title imbued with the optimistic view that you will continue living beyond its temporary usage. The general indications are that you would like a.) everything possible done to keep you alive, b.) nothing done, unless a fall and rapid recovery is assumed or, c.) something in the middle. Most people don't know that you can specify details like "I never want electric shocks" or "I never want to be fed through a tube in my stomach." Sometimes this makes people feel they have more control over their lives and bodies in the midst of debilitating illness. Still, the word "power" might catch you as it does me. How ironic that a document that seems to grant authority is invoked just when we feel the most powerless.

The bottom line, however, is that even in this era of high-tech medicine none of us—no matter how familiar we may be with the US medical system—can foresee all possible combinations and permutations of a person's medical reality. This is why it is so important to identify someone to be your surrogate—your POA. Remember, that person has absolutely no authority as long as you are alert and well oriented. And you can change your POA simply by crossing out the old name and replacing it with a new one. Just be sure to initial and date the change. If you haven't completed a POA for yourself, you might want to consider it. I know that it seems inconsequential in the midst of all you are going through. I hope that you will fill out one of those little forms for yourself as you are sitting at the bedside. You are surely seeing in a whole new way how important it is to have someone who understands your healthy self to come alongside you when you are ill. You should *have the same tender care at the end of your life that you yourself are providing in these days.*

Choosing a medical POA warrants some serious thought. The person you pick is not necessarily the person you love the most or the one you would not want to offend or your firstborn child. The person you select should be someone who knows better than anyone else what sort of medical care you would like in a critical situation. That person should also be strong enough to carry out your wishes, even if their own personal desires are different from yours, and even under the pressure they may experience from relatives or friends. It is a tough job. Well, I suppose you know that if you've already faced the reality of being identified as your husband's POA. It is a tremendous privilege and an equally tremendous responsibility. Don't be afraid to ask questions as they arise—as many as you need to ask. Don't be afraid to include the doctors in your decision making. They not only help you when they join you in these conversations, but they also gain clarity regarding the sort of treatment that patients might elect.

The responsibility of being Dennis's POA weighs heavily on me during his final ten days, but I would never cede my role to another human being. I have no doubt at all about what sort of care Dennis wants at the end of his life. We have discussed countless scenarios when he was very alert and certainly well oriented. We talked about the progress of his disease as he experienced it and what his fears were for the future. Some days our conversations and his journal entries centered on his fear that he was dying. Other times his deeper anxiety was that his symptoms' crescendo had nothing to do with life expectancy. The thought that he was destined to live decades in this tortured body truly terrified him more than anything else.

Every day has come to be a house of horrors through which Dennis somehow finds his way. No matter how much I love him and commit myself to being present with him during these dark days, the truth is stark: there are places—"tricky, treacherous, and mean" as Dennis described them—that none of us who love him can go. I used to fantasize about taking turns with Dennis, inhabiting his body for a time so he could enjoy the freedoms of mine. How I wished I could gift him with a plunge into the ocean waves, a chance to attack the moguls once more on a black-diamond ski run, or even the simple satisfaction of helping one of our kids move into a new apartment.

My wishes in these moments exceeded Dennis's wildest dreams. He fixated on less glorious hopes. When he was still able to travel for his work, he would have paid dearly to be able to board a plane without panicking when the fasten seatbelt sign lit up because he knew his legs would scream their horrendous cacophony of pain if he could not get up and move around. Not being able to shovel the snow in our driveway drove him crazy, since Mr. Gallant believed that this was his God-given responsibility. He felt constrained by waves of fatigue that left him as something less than the life of the party—a whole new experience for Mr. Fun. But as the disease continued its insidious march, skiing and travel and parties teased him less often. Each day had more primal longings. Dennis just wanted to be able to dress himself and cut his own toenails. He wanted to drink water without choking. He would have liked to write his thoughts in his journal without dropping the pen repeatedly. As much as I observe and as hard as I listen, I don't think I will ever fully grasp the perverse paradox he lived: the more dependent people become on others, the more likely they are to be relationally isolated.

As we hole up in this hospital room, I become more and more committed to cocooning my husband in the adoration of our marriage, hoping to make the "for worse" just a little bit better. I instinctively know that this is the end-of-life equivalent of a honeymoon. We are alone together in a room for a week. In stark contrast to the previous year's inpatient hospice stay when people came in droves to sit by Dennis's bedside, there are no visitors this time. Everyone should have their dearest family and friends fly in to say goodbye—once. We need a new strategy. In the game of life, this is overtime, and I am the quarterback. Dennis is so deeply committed to his many relationships that, until now, when teetering precariously on the edge of life, he would expend his dwindling reserves of energy to connect with his visitors. Now Dennis cannot interact with anyone, and I am certainly in no position to entertain guests. I want to focus exclusively on my dying husband. There will be time for me to merge back into community life. The reality that we have an army of people wanting to support us is surely part of the reason I am able to bear this temporary isolation. This time is sacred.

I am well supported in guarding this sacred space by many on the hospital staff. One of these is Jennifer Clark, who was assigned as Dennis's RN for some early days and then rearranged her schedule—even a day off—so that she could be with him as much as possible. I will be forever grateful for her kindnesses to me as well as her care of Dennis. She did things like offer to chart from the computer in his room while I e-mailed friends in another space. She encouraged me to get outside for quick walks. She asked if I was eating enough. When I tease her about being our "nurse angel," something in my brain clicks, and I ask, "Isn't that a song?"

"No, I don't think so."

I start humming and we realize simultaneously that I am thinking of "Earth Angel." While we are laughing and singing, my minimally responsive husband pipes in! It is just a few notes, but they are precious.

Jennifer is, however, at her most angelic when she speaks with our daughter, Brittany. I thought that our two girls understood the gravity of their dad's medical situation. What I had forgotten is that it is difficult to sustain the sense of urgency over fourteen months when an illness moves from chronic to acute to imminent. Brittany is planning an out-of-state trip with college friends.

"Britt, Dad is not doing well. I am not sure you should go so far away."

"Mom! You said that last year!" She accuses me and dismisses me simultaneously.

"I know this has been a long year…"

"I want to speak with Dad's doctor." It is late in the day, and I do not expect to see another MD until the morning.

"Would you like to speak to his nurse?" Jennifer is in the room and overhears me. She feigns horror but takes the receiver from me. She explains that Dennis is displaying end-of-life symptoms but cautions that no one can predict when a person will die. She somehow cushions the truth. This suffices to corral Brittany's emotions. Love tethers her to Dennis while fear pulls her away. The delicate tension is restored, and Brittany and I are able to speak candidly.

While my senses are taking in as much as they can, my mind is formulating a little pen-and-ink book of illustrations, entitled *Fifty Ways to Configure Hospital Furniture*. Whenever Dennis is positioned in such a way that my own body might not disturb his, I climb into the bed with him. The electronically regulated mattress ebbs and flows like the tide in a benevolent attempt to protect Dennis's skin from bedsores, but at times it seems to swallow him up. I contort myself with considerable creativity around that bed. I find I can slide the monstrosity on its casters and prop myself up by Dennis's side. Using the wall, a small, straight-backed chair, and a standard-issue green plastic recliner, I drape myself alongside the man I have shared a bed with for nearly twenty-five years. As the disease process devours my Dennis, I want more and more to be near him. I want to be sure that I hear anything he might say, and I do not want him to be without companionship on this last bit of life. I wind myself around my props in some pretty odd ways and delight in being close to him.

The present is all I can see, but the expanse of time I will come to know as my very own AD—After Dennis—looms furtively on the horizon. I anticipate moments piled high like blocks or strung long like beads or scattered wide by grief when I will long for the privilege of being in the same physical space as my husband. I spend these days absorbing all I can in preparation for those when recall will be all I have. I try to commit his physical essence to memory by systematically studying him. I run my hand down his arms and lock my fingers in his limp hand. I play with his wedding band until I eventually soap it liberally and slide it from his finger to my own. I trace the contours of his face with my nose. I put my lips lightly to his and linger for what seems like a very long time. I want to remember how soft they are. I want to remember their thin sweetness and how I have always said that he has "sinister lips," which made him laugh with decidedly not-sinister delight. I cup his kneecaps. The hair on his calves is matted with sweat and lotion, and I make it my project to smooth it out. I find settling places for my head: the crook of his elbow, the back of his neck, the pit of his arm, and the soft side of his waist. I stay still and enjoy each spot in a way that was not possible when Dennis was more alert and being touched exacerbated his pain. When he moves—and he invariably does—I pull back and let him recalibrate his bizarre body before I move in again. I find myself breathing abnormally. Sometimes I catch myself beginning to hyperventilate as I take in the reality that my husband is actively dying. More often, I take deep breaths from his bedside and hold them in my lungs. I definitely inhale.

We are alone in a room suspended in a world with no regard for clock time or social propriety. It is not unusual for hospital staff to stop by at 10:00 p.m. to review some aspect of Dennis's care or arrive at 4:30 a.m. to shave him. All we have invested in one another is culminating in the space between us. Not only is Dennis dying, but our marriage—a separate thing—is coming to its final denouement. Just as we packed our bags in anticipation of our honeymoon, we arrived at the hospital with a few of our belongings: shirts and boxers and slippers and khakis that would be worn for twenty-four-hour days under comfortable tops, an iPod and knitting and the old leather shaving kit I gave Dennis early in our marriage. A friend has sent my favorite wine, complete with corkscrew. It is a lovely gesture, and yes, I drink it alone as evenings slide into nights and nothing else changes.

Early in the hospitalization, when Dennis was alert enough to eat, we shared his meal tray—the Jell-O, not the creamed soups. I have always picked food off his plate in restaurants; it somehow tastes better than whatever I have ordered. But this is not a practice he finds endearing. After a couple of decades of irritation, Dennis finally asked me with some measure of consternation, "You're really not trying to stop eating off my plate, are you?"

The question surprised me, but I faced it head-on: "No. I figure it gives me more pleasure than it gives you displeasure." Then it was his turn to be surprised. But thankfully, he did not challenge my functional premise and accepted my annoying habit as a fact of life. We share in the hospital, and he does not comment. When he can no longer share, I eat the food alone.

That is about the same time I start using his toothbrush. It is there in the bathroom, sticking out of the shaving kit I packed. I am looking at myself in the mirror as I wash my face and slip into Dennis's T-shirt and boxers for the night. I am talking to myself. This is not a product of my anxious grief; I have been talking to myself since I was a kid. As I brush my teeth with his toothbrush, I tell myself that Dennis and I, in some ways, have never been so close. Here we are physically tethered as I find new ways to curl around him in his bed, but we are also intellectually and emotionally bonded as thoughts and feelings surrounding his impending death fill every part of my being. I am keenly aware that, now that he is rarely conscious and would certainly never pass for "decisional," I am Dennis's functional decision-maker, his POA. I reason that if I can make end-of-life decisions for Dennis, I can use his toothbrush. But even as I justify my pilfering the toothbrush, I weep at the realization that he will never make another decision about his world again. Not about all those complex medical decisions that shroud end-of-life and not about his toothbrush.

TALKING POINTS FOR MORTALS

1. Do you have a Health Care Power of Attorney document prepared?
2. Who among your loved ones best understand - or at least accepts - your health care preferences generally and especially around end of life care?
3. Have you asked this person - and others? - to advocate for you in the event that you become unable to do that for yourself?

■ ■ ■

CHAPTER 6

Pain

[peyn] n. physical suffering variously described by quality, location, and intensity

Most medical interaction in a US hospital now includes the question, "On a scale of zero to ten, with ten being the most severe pain that you can imagine, how would you rate your pain?" The answer is noted with the presumption that the patient's perceptions have been honored. For Dennis, this methodology didn't register an accurate read. Not even close. Dennis was a man of generous spirit who had grown up in the middle of a large, middle-class family. He was scrappy. He was tough. He had a high tolerance for pain. If he got tackled, he came back. If he fell on a ski slope, he got right back up to conquer the offending moguls with a vengeance. Before this horrendous disease took up residence in Dennis's body, he had never missed a day of work. Never. Complaining wasn't part of his vocabulary, and whining simply wasn't an option.

Initially, as his illness took root through small starts and large fits, Dennis puzzled at the question, "On a scale of zero to ten, with ten being the most severe pain that you can imagine, how would you rate your pain?"

"Relative to what?" he would ask me. "What kind of pain are they talking about?"

It took being half way to hell before he ever sought medical attention for what was happening in his body. But when he finally acknowledged that his pain was extraordinary, he saw a doctor who asked him to rate it. Dennis started with a five, probably for lack of any better guess. Eventually he seemed to get the hang of the question. As the disease became increasingly intrusive, he gave progressively higher numbers. Until he got to eight. Even though I could plainly see behaviors and journal entries indicating increasing pain, Dennis stuck with eight. When it was staggeringly plain that things were getting worse, he ceded to an eight and a half. And after months of Dennis claiming to be eight and a half and holding, his unbearable, untreatable pain drove him to admit himself to the hospital for palliative sedation for the second time in fourteen months. Yet, even in this final desperation, Dennis would not give a higher number no matter by whom or how often the question was posed.

Dennis's reasoning was that a nine would be what he had witnessed in the births of his two precious baby girls—both accompanied by protracted back labor. Even as his life was slipping away and the conversation was supposed to be centered on his extraordinary pain, he found a way to honor me. Amazingly charming. It was, however, not so useful for Dennis or his medical team as they considered how to treat his pain. Obviously, if he couldn't get to a nine, he could not even contemplate a ten. I had to challenge him on this because, from where I sat, it sure looked like Dennis was living in a skin that he would give anything to unzip and crawl out of. He looked surprised by my prompting and clung even tighter to his stoic stance. "If you're able to say 'ten,' you can't be experiencing the worst imaginable pain."

So much for nominal scales.

There is also the matter of Dennis's perennial optimism that caused me such consternation during the initial hospital admission assessment. It just is not Dennis's nature to paint a grim picture of his own need. Instead, he talks himself through each bout with despair by searching for the life lesson his struggles present. Although he would not have been foolish enough to choose this suffering, he is sage enough to embrace it. As a result, the depth and breadth of his compassion for others increases incrementally with his pain. The transformation is evident. I wonder if these strategies might be, to some degree, acts of self-preservation motivated by the subconscious. What I mean is that, perhaps if the pain were unnamed, it might be kept from being untamed. If the notion that "things could be worse" began as a defense mechanism, it later proves a dreadful portent laden with fear.

Nothing frightens Dennis more than the possibility that the pain will continue its infiltration of systems and senses faster than he can adjust to it. And he has good reason to be very frightened. I am frightened. I am trying to be professional about my role as this man's advocate but I adore him, and that is not terribly professional. Dennis's life becomes more and more untenable as pain overtakes him. At some point, I begin to make peace with a strange comfort: my husband will not be forever trapped in a body of unremitting and truly unbearable pain because, ultimately, my husband will die from this disease. I know that for months he has met the Medicare criteria for hospice admission, which means that with natural disease progression he is not expected to live more than six months. The same cruel malady that wrought this suffering will eventually bring it to an end. I cannot imagine that it will take long now, but of course, "long" is a relative term.

As I watch this man who personifies courage and tenacity crumble, I find myself embracing a new thought: it will be good when Dennis dies. Of course I do not share this with anyone, not even Dennis at first. But soon, our talks about heaven and its promise of a new glorified body bring us both comfort rather than anxiety. The stark reality of what is happening to Dennis has forced us to explore intellectual and emotional territory that healthy people rarely tread. As a direct result of these conversations, I have a sense that Dennis and I share a special space of intimacy that I would neither wish on anyone nor trade for anything in the world. Except perhaps a miraculous healing.

If the goal of this chapter is to help you, dear Other Wife, to think of pain more broadly as you go through the struggle with your beloved, I must share how Dennis's pain impacts me. In the context of our profoundly deep love, it is the pain that enables me not only to let Dennis go, but also to help him go. It surprises even me (and many of our friends) that I have no inclination to cling to him and thus prolong the dying process. I want Dennis to know that he has invested in me and in our girls and in our extended family and in our precious friends beyond measure. It is time for him to be at rest. I truly want him to be ushered respectfully from this place of torture and despair. So I embrace without any hesitation the privilege of working with the palliative care team to accomplish what is referred to as a "good death" or "dying well." This does not mean that I don't ache at the prospect of living the rest of my life without my Dennis. It does not mean that I have made peace with the notion of being a forty-seven-year-old widow. I can only begin to imagine the loss that our daughters will suffer, both now and as their lives unfold. But right now the world is reduced to one hospital room. As Dennis's wife, his POA, I am wholeheartedly committed to the privilege of prayerfully escorting him to the end of this temporal life.

Dennis was brutally honest about his pain in the journal he kept through the darkness of his illness. For three years he quite literally hosted pain day and night. There were moments when he was able to dance with it. Mostly he wrestled. Sometimes he wept. I can think of no better way to illustrate what brought us to this hospitalization than to share Dennis's own words from his journal:

I need to focus and push through. I feel like I am behind in everything I do. So I really need to kick it into gear even though I feel like my gears are stripped. (September 2005)

I'm not sure how this is going to go from here—but it's not looking good. There must be something to be done—but I'm not sure what. I will call my doctor tonight. (February 2006)

I think about killing myself on days like this and almost curse the fact that I have all these reasons to live. Mostly my Susan, Brittany, and Juliana need me. Also, I have always regarded suicide as a cowardly and selfish act. (May 2006)

I feel so unfailingly miserable that I run the risk of falling into depression. I often muse about dying. I can't imagine living another thirty to thirty-five years like this. Ultimately I think my body would just quit. But for now I'd like to have a physical hope as well as a spiritual hope. I need to develop some real goals to keep my focus—to keep active—to keep my sense of humor. (July 2006)

This has been a dark and difficult day emotionally. The unrelenting aspect of the disease attack is particularly maddening. Sometimes I have this suffering thing down. Other times I am just frustrated. It is difficult to write. (August 2006)

I always feel lousy despite the new therapies. She [the MD] challenged me to see a shrink...I'm not sure what to do with that. Do I feel awful? Yes.

Do I get discouraged with that? Yes. Do I have dark times when I feel like taking a swan dive out of the office window? Yes, absolutely. But I also have a strong faith in my Lord. (August 2006)

So much for the pithy words of friends who say things like, "It will work out okay." No, sometimes it really doesn't. Sometimes life is just a big mess. (October 2006)

I am CONSTANTLY thinking about my disease! It ALWAYS has a grip on me. (March 2007)

I believe I have turned a comer...I believe I have learned more about how to suffer. I really want to be the man who was described by Thomas à Kempis in his classic, *Imitation of Christ*: "Whoever best knows how to suffer will keep the greatest peace. That man is a conqueror of himself." (June 2007)

My disease elbows its way into every moment, reminding me of its presence—gnawing away at the inclination I might have to rest, relax, and enjoy (July 2007).

It is very difficult to get ready—shave and shower—and especially get dressed. It's hard to take the train. It is increasingly difficult to walk from the train to my office. It is hard to sit, and it is hard to stand. My bowels and bladder wreak havoc...I am tired of putting a good face on things...I need to constantly be brave. Getting out of bed requires bravery. I need to be brave to flee thoughts of taking my own life. (August 2007)

At times my unrelenting pain makes me feel like I am drowning while someone has a fire hose trained on me. The emotional darkness that this brings is utterly stunning. I have experienced grief and blackness and emotional loneliness, hopelessness and despair that were far beyond anything that I ever imagined. Processing the grief while in very pitched levels of pain seemed impossible. Suicide [sic] ideation involves trying to dig yourself out of a hole by calling on all your resources to avoid going there. The decision to commit suicide involves a surreal disorientation. Choosing death seems to be like choosing to breathe…

My body is such a confluence of pain and dysfunction. This notion of looking good is also a problem with all my doctors. They have no %#$%#*@* idea how hard this is. They work with pain patients and so the think they know. But they are clueless. I can tell by their questions, by their responses, and by their "deer in the headlights" expression when I am speaking with them. And I fear their clinical notes. Any discouraging word from my mouth and I get labeled "depressed." I suppose they don't have a category from their clinical training that quite captures the notion that their patient has intelligently assessed the treatment they are receiving, and in the judgment of the patient, the doctor has been found wanting. Lacking such a classification, the clinician marks the patient as "depressed"—and they are on to the next patient. (April 2008)

I am overwhelmed with grief. My losses continue to pile up. My ability to do any physical tasks

continues to decline. My pain is relentless and excruciating. (May 2008)

It is difficult to overstate the existential pain that such
physical pain spawns. For three years Dennis got out of bed
each day committed to putting one foot in front of the
other, hoping to live rather than just survive. I still marvel at
his resolve. As closely as I watch this man, help where I can,
and pray where I cannot, I am confident that I would be
stunned if I could experience firsthand the physical realities
of his days.

As Dennis's body becomes more and more limited, and
even more racked by pain, something deep within his soul
rises to meet it. The spiritual experiences are precious and
sweet and certainly hard earned. To these Dennis clings like
the desperate man he is. In an e-mail message designed to
comfort his youngest sister, Kate, Dennis wrote:

> As to the meaning of suffering...knowing the mean-
> ing does make it far more bearable. Our Lord does
> use (if we submit) suffering as an instrument to
> lead us on the path to becoming more like Jesus...
> and to really know and enjoy his presence. This is a
> very mysterious Truth. I am staggered by the relent-
> lessness of my suffering, but I am doing far better
> emotionally and spiritually even as my health dete-
> riorates further.

In another e-mail sent to a longer list of family and
friends just twelve days before he died, Dennis wrote:

A few weeks ago my pain jumped to a new level… One of my doctors thinks I am some rare genetic freak that can withstand pain at an incredible level. I beg to differ…Finding peace, experiencing joy, and remaining hopeful are great challenges…but for me, it always comes back to Jesus. In the midst of my misery, I strain into Him and find solace there.

As I watch Dennis lose his orientation to all but the body he has battled for three years, I am a woman bifurcated. My husband as I have known him is disappearing. Grief would overwhelm me but for the concurrent reality that my husband's disease will soon have none of its proverbial sting. I long for Dennis to be released from his pain. To that end, I embrace my charge as his end-of-life companion. Whatever decisions I make in his stead are for the express intention of minimizing his short- and long-term discomfort. I am not afraid to ask for clarity around every procedure and potion and probe. I am not going to let anything or anyone add to Dennis's suffering. Not on my watch.

In the midst of a delirious oration of about half a dozen isolated words thrown out into the room, Dennis is finally uninhibited enough to express what I know he has experienced for months, if not years:

"Ten."

TALKING POINTS FOR MORTALS

1. Do you understand what pain is anticipated in your illness as it progresses?
2. What is your experience of pain in other contexts? How does that experience impact your life?
3. How might you be as specific as possible with your medical team regarding how you feel and how you would like to be treated generally and medicated specifically?

■ ■ ■

CHAPTER 7

Music

[myoo-zik] n. art of organizing complex sound in temporal relationship for accompaniment and pleasure

Music is something rudimentary and raw for Dennis. He is always the man with a song, not the one just enjoying music. From our earliest dates Dennis would blast the car stereo, use the seat belt as an impromptu guitar and croon to me, screech at me, or quiz me. For him, listening to the radio was an interactive game.

"Do you know who's singing?"

"What year?"

"Do you know the *original* title?"

"Who did the backup?"

I failed all the quizzes. They were rigged. Dennis would just keep asking questions until I was stumped. Sometimes that meant he had to ask more than one. Usually not. It amused him to no end, and that, in turn, amused me. We had our act down.

On this bright, sunny fifth day of hospitalization, Dennis comes out of his stupor and makes a full, if brief, appearance. He presents just the way you would expect a man to present after a disease-fueled, drug-induced, four-day nap. (Think Rip van Winkle in a blue-green hospital gown.) He has not been shaved for a couple of days. The mix of bedding and fever-sweat that comes with illness mats his hair. His teeth have acquired a soapy film and seem to have grown too large for his mouth. It is not a jolted wakening of any urgency. Rather, Dennis just eases back to me. He moves more frequently and more expansively. He opens his eyes and focuses first on my face and then on his surroundings. He speaks unintelligibly at first, on and off for a couple of hours. Then he speaks like Dennis:

"Do you have my iPod?"

I do, of course. No one who knows Dennis and really loves him would separate the man from his music. I put in his earbuds.

"What would you like to hear?" I ask. But before he can answer, he drifts back into that space I cannot share. I select Springsteen for him, one of many surrogate decisions I make as he moves from "we" to that place that is more and more just "I." He emerges again a few hours later and seems to know that he has been absent for some of, as he says, "all the news that's fit to print," and so he sends me out in search of the *New York Times*. As I set off, I remember the day about a year ago when Dennis began to see that he was becoming disoriented by his disease and its remedies, exacerbated by the hospital setting he was in. He said with absolutely no hint of humor, "How do they expect me to get oriented if I don't have Cheerios, black coffee, and the *New York Times* at the beginning of the day?" As I recall that daily ritual, I think of the friends over time who have observed with awe just how much this slight man eats every morning. (Three large bowls of Multigrain Cheerios topped with granola). But knowing these details of everyday life, and honoring them, can make all the difference.

This day doesn't bring any major care plan changes. This is partially due to the fact that hospitals move to a different rhythm on weekends. Staffing is thin. Care plan changes deemed something less than emergent are delayed to involve more collegial input where that is an option. For Dennis, this is a day of more resting. For me the day is marked by greater stillness and increasing intensity. Dennis is markedly less alert today. As he disappears, I feel a responsibility to be attentive to a commensurate degree. In the middle of this day, Dennis pops back for few words...a smile...a funny face intended to elicit a giggle from me. Somehow—there is *no way* that there isn't a great and mighty sovereign God in our midst—Dennis's hospital room is quiet and peaceful. I ask our friends and even family to refrain from arriving to punctuate this experience. Dennis cannot entertain and in fact is in this place for the specific goal of sedation. I'm committed to soaking up as much of him as I possibly can. Clear as I am about this plan, I'm surprised by my own serenity. It's not boring to just sit and be with Dennis. It's not scary. It's not lonely. It is simply a privilege, and I am blown away by the special graces held for me in this space.

I'm thinking of you, Other Wife, and I'm praying that you find this sweet spot too. It's a place made precious in part because it's such a scarce commodity. Time together just doing life cannot be taken for granted anymore. How incredibly improbable is my sense of peace! I suspect that these days will forever be sprinkled with fairy dust in my mind. I know that soon I will long for their intimate luxury: two lovers alone with nothing but the breath of life between them...

Music has always been part of Dennis. He has a lovely voice and an uncanny memory for lyrics. But it's the nuance of a song that Dennis has down to an art form. He can make it rise and swell and can use it to still anyone from a fussy child to a petulant adult—usually me. What woman wouldn't melt to her own personalized version of "Calendar Girl" or when listening to her husband entertain a room full of friends? One of our friends tells of a wedding reception we attended where Dennis taught an original arrangement of a couple of love songs to serenade the bride and groom. When our daughters were infants, he used familiar melodies and created his own one-of-a-kind lullaby for each of them. Brittany's song talked about how *tiny* our precious baby seemed to him. Juliana's brimmed with his delight that she "came to stay."

It is the loss of song—the day the music dies—that produces the first distinct gnawing in my gut. I realize that I have always counted on Dennis to make life sing. My contribution in our marriage has been to set the tone, to measure the beat, to guard the rhythm. But it's Dennis who gives the song its life. As Dennis's disease progresses the music quite naturally changes, and eventually fades to distant echoes. Like the shelter of a shadow, the echoes have come to have their own special service.

I'm not the first person won over by Dennis's songs. At his memorial service both of his younger sisters told of their brother serenading them: "Old songs: Ricky Nelson, Scott McKenzie; Crosby, Stills, Nash & Young...Sweet songs: 'I love to see cottonwood blossoms in the early spring...'" MaryAnne recalled.

"He had a remarkable memory for lyrics...He would sing every word of 'Mr. Tambourine Man,' 'American Pie,' and 'Bobby McGee,'" reported Kate. She also got some laughs pointing out that their other brothers—four of them—would say, "Don't get him started."

I understood that caution; it was much easier to turn the music on than it was to tune it out. Dennis was a man of temperance in many areas. Song was not one of them. I will forever be grateful for the myriad ways that he constructed a soundtrack for our lives together. He did passionate renditions of love songs—yes, that is 75 percent of what is out there—while I did our bookkeeping. He sang rebellious, edgy lyrics from the Vietnam era just when our girls might have thought we understood *nothing* of the real world of high school in the twenty-first century. Dennis pulled out old spirituals while he cleaned up the kitchen after friends had left our dinner table. The veins in his neck protruded when he belted out Bruce Springsteen, his favorite rock 'n' roll poet. Sweet smile lines cradled his renditions of Chris

Tomlin and Caedman's Call. He found new meaning in the songs Warren Zevon sang at the end of his life. But mostly, the music was Dennis's prop. At times, the music was so central that Dennis himself seemed to be the prop.

Lest I leave you with the impression that it was always romantic to live with Mr. Music, I admit to some discordant moments. Early in our relationship I needed to help Dennis understand that when I was expressing my annoyance over some aspect of his existence or its intersection with mine, it was not acceptable to respond with a song lyric. Every happily married couple will admit to some issues that keep coming up. My eating food off his plate was one. His singing to me when I was irritated was another. I don't always agree to dance to his music. But he never stops trying to make me.

Even when disease had robbed Dennis of the ability to sing well—and he did have a sweet, clear tenor voice—he would cue up some cut and jack the stereo so that wherever I was or whatever I was doing, I was forced to meet him in the lyric of his moment. That, or just be irritated by the volume as I tried to ignore it. I would find my way to where he stood—invariably beside the tuner near his desk. Better to respond to his summons and to sway with him in what had become a poor imitation of the junior high shuffle. Better to remember that I was married to a man who wanted to share all of life's songs with me, even when those songs were increasingly downbeat and frighteningly morose. As Dennis was increasingly crippled, when I arrived and stood before him, he would push off from the desk he had invariably been using to hold himself upright. His weak arms would arc in unison from the edge of the desk onto my shoulders. He would shift and redistribute his weight forward until his chest barreled into mine. By hooking my arms under his armpits, I could be a reliable prop, strong enough to last the few minutes of a CD track. Dennis would have already lowered the lights. He would close his eyes. I don't honestly know where he went when we danced. He didn't talk or laugh or twirl me around as he had for most of our marriage when we had been surrounded by music either recorded or rendered by Dennis himself. These dances were more a part of a journey he invited me to share than a moment of levity we enjoyed. That said, I counted it a privilege to be invited to go to this musical holding place with him. I would breathe in the smell of his sweater and his neck. I would notice how his increasingly weak frame would drape over me. There was one night just days before his last hospitalization when it dawned on me that I was almost carrying him to the music. It was evocative. I was not sure of exactly what.

Dennis's musical preferences were not changing as much as they were taking on a different hue. During his last year of life, Dennis found recordings that Johnny Cash made in the six-month period between when June Carter Cash died and when he followed her from this earth. He listened to more and more music that was downbeat and in minor keys. His singing was less and less musical and lilting and more and more raspy and ragged. Juliana referred to the new repertoire as "Dad's death music." I tried to get her off that track because I found the implications upsetting. But in fact she was right. Dennis's siblings and I understood that some of these lyrics had simply been internalized as art with which he could resonate. These artists' struggles with their own versions of the existential dilemma gave Dennis a vehicle for his own expression. Kate would tell of the sick feeling that washed over her when she realized that Dennis's singing into the phone "My Ride Is Here" was his way of telling his little sister that he would not be with her on this earth much longer. Brittany would recall how very often she heard her Dad sing to me, "and should I fall behind, wait for me," as we drove around doing errands. Brittany would also be brave enough—would also be Dennis enough—to sing for those gathered at his memorial service about how her dad was Nat-King-Cole unforgettable. People asked me how she could find and hold her voice at such a time. My standard response in the days after the memorial service was, "I haven't a clue." I later revised my answer: "She's her daddy's girl." Brittany had been rehearsing for her whole life and one evening.

Virtually anything associated with Dennis is a vein from which I can draw life. In this time when Dennis's death seems increasingly nigh, I look up and realize that I miss the music. Terribly. The phrase "the day the music died," although attributed to someone else, now has a special resonance. I miss the lightening of tensions that the tunes allow. I miss the intensity of the lyrics that Dennis demands I strain to catch. (He wrote many of them out for me when I failed). I start playing his iPod for myself and running his CDs. I relish the handwritten papers on which he has scrawled those lyrics. I sing to him and for him and because of him. It makes me cry. And that feels good too.

While Dennis's special twist on life can be understood through a discussion of music, it's not the music that matters. Whatever matters most to you is what matters. Music is here intended to include facets of the beloved's soul. Of his or her essential nature.

I think of you, Other Wife, when the music plays on Dennis's iPod and I know that I have been able to bring a little bit of our more normal lives into this place where Dennis will die. I want you to be able to focus on the person in the bed. Not just the bed with your dear person in it. And it's awfully easy to let the hospitalization at end of life take on a life of its own—a life that overtakes the person being treated. You don't want to lose the uniqueness of your beloved one minute before death is pronounced. I suppose you don't really ever want to lose the person you adore. In the weeks and months and years to come, the horrors of this vigil will fade and be replaced by clearer images of your real life together. That's what all the bereavement literature promises. I'm holding onto that research tightly for both our sakes. The hospital is just the setting. Don't let it consume the person you love.

I keep trying to think of facets of Dennis's life that I can bring to the hospital to keep that space from swallowing him up. Some people put blown-up photographs of people they love on the walls to remind professional staff that this person in the bed has a real life and real relationships. Other people like to keep a TV or radio tuned to a favorite channel. Many like to tell stories to anyone who will listen. All of these are ways of protecting the person as long as his or her heart is beating. I consider it my role in large part to interpret my husband's unique essence to the professionals caring for Dennis, lest he be lost to the process of receiving that care.

"His face is always ruddy," I remind them.

"The horizontal lines just above the bridge of his nose knot when he is in excruciating pain," I explain.

"He's more uncomfortable leaning on his right hip."

"He likes to be clean shaven."

"No, the choking is not new."

One of my last roles as Mrs. Dennis Patrick Sheehan is to interpret a dying man's language. A language he now speaks without words. As Dennis's beautiful voice falls silent, my voice will have to suffice. So I choose my words carefully and measure them out as faithfully as I know how.

TALKING POINTS FOR MORTALS

1. What gives you the greatest and most unbridled crazy-wonderful joy?
2. How can this joy be preserved as your illness progress? How might it change as your illness progresses?

∎ ∎ ∎

CHAPTER 8

Palliation

[pal-ee-ey-shuhn] n. interdisciplinary attempt to address distressing symptoms rather than mitigate their source

F ew people get a rehearsal for their last days of life on earth. Dennis did. Fifteen months before this last hospitalization, he was admitted for a month of care at an inpatient hospice for what was then considered a "pain crisis." Indeed it was. At that time Dennis's life expectancy was not clear; professional estimates ranged from days to years. Those are odd things to hear. I found it difficult to get my emotional brain around the notion that this could be a sprint to death or a marathon decline. Toggling back and forth between the two has its own special challenges.

How do we pace ourselves when we don't know how far we have to go, dear Other Wife? You'll find that just as you settle into one routine, your role will demand that you adopt another.

Without a clue of what this prognosis meant, I relayed the facts and encouraged anyone who was able and so inclined to visit. In order to be responsible to Dennis's sprawling extended family and especially to our daughters who were both in college, I had to warn them that time could be short. Friends were dispatched to meet the girls at their respective colleges, give them this information, and help get them home. Loved ones came from across the country to visit Dennis and offered what support they could for our girls and me. They cooked, catered, did laundry, and supplied us with CDs, red wine, Black Label, and expressions and tokens of their commitment to walk this part of our lives with us in the context of community. In the fifteen months since that time, we have lived the long good-bye, and I am as exhausted as I am grieved.

> *I can't help but note, Other Wife, that this is the same thing we're being told now, over a year later. But this time I'm sure that we are in Dennis's final days even if the medical professionals are still uncertain. A wife knows what a wife knows.*

"Everyone should have a send-off at the end of their life like you did, Dream Man," I told my precious husband about a month before this last hospitalization. "Once." He knew I was serious. It had taken me much of the intervening year to recover from "entertaining" the throngs of people who wanted some time with Dennis. A month of sixteen-hour days crammed with ever-increasing amounts of relational interaction and emotional investment into these wonderful people had worn me out. We had moved from the house where we raised our family to a handicapped-accessible town home, I was working full time as a hospice social worker, and, more weekends than not, we hosted out-of-state guests.

But this season is different. Most notably, Dennis is much sicker and can't even attempt to entertain visitors. He can no longer communicate verbally, even with me. Aside from that, one of the primary medical goals of this hospitalization is to medicate Dennis to a point where he loses awareness of his pain. Dennis needs quiet and calm above all else this time around, but there's no precedent for such solitude in this man's history. Dennis warned me. When we were engaged and considering honeymoon options, he admitted that he "couldn't imagine spending a whole week with just one person." Not the best words to toss at a bride-to-be! As it turns out, he did just fine alone with me for a week, and we had a good story to share after that glorious escape.

So this time, it's no visitors. I need to concentrate my energy on being the best sojourner for Dennis. If there is anything I can do to make him even incrementally more comfortable, I want to be available. I am steadily trained on him. I know that Dennis's life and our marriage are winding down. I know that there will be countless times when I will want just one more smell of his face, a touch of his arm, a gaze at his neck, and the taste of his lips. I am committed to stockpiling against the inevitable. I think of these days as a time to soak in as much of my husband as I possibly can.

As my visceral self fills itself with tender memories of Dennis, my intellectual self readies itself for battle. I am determined to advocate not only for my husband, but for all patients in need of palliative care in this prestigious teaching hospital better known for allopathic care and its commitment to aggressive investment in cure. I would relish a cure, to be sure. But if there is none, the distinction between prolonging life and protracting death becomes crucial. I'm not thinking that I will spend the rest of Dennis's hospitalization lobbying for what my professional and personal experience convinces me is best for end-of-life patients.

At some point on this day of my vigil, I realize that I will not hear my husband speak again. I rifle through the last days measured in horrific hours punctuated by excruciating moments searching for his last words. Dennis's voice has always soothed me. It really doesn't matter what he says, although he has always lavished me with kind words. It is just a quality he has. But now the combination of disease progression and medical intervention pulls Dennis to some distant realm. His voice has aged in sync with the rest of his physical self. I still cling to his words. But they changed too. Until Dennis's illness dragged us through thirty years of aging in three, I noticed that the stereotypic rigid, cautious, and formal speech patterns of the elderly ran parallel to physical decline. Now I am coming to see how interconnected they are—how the physical sensation of aging demands a different sort of speech. Fear of being unable to cope with the physical demands of life led Dennis to be purposeful in his activities rather than spontaneous. Formal speech patterns reflected the awareness that we would not have the rest of our lives to say what needed to be said. In the last few months of Dennis's life, I've been stunned at the changes in his social behavior. For the first time in our marriage, I lived with a man who was easily sated by relationships. He drew his social circle closer. He struggled to get past the physical realities of his disease to engage people at a deeper level. He desperately fought the tendency of being self-centered.

Privately Dennis took to holding my face between his two familiarly square hands that now shook slightly. Looking deep into my eyes, like you might expect of a man who does not expect to have the opportunity much longer, he would say, "You are *so* dear to me," and, "I could not have asked for anything more in a wife". The words were uttered with an old man's syntax and invariably accompanied by a distant smile or a reassuring pat. Initially, I wasn't sure what to make of these expressions of love. But I've come to treasure them for what I suspect they are: part of a conscientiously selected repertoire intended to carry me though the parts of life stretching before me that we both know I will live as Dennis Patrick Sheehan's widow. It dawns on me, sitting in this hospital and remembering his intentionality, that while some will say that Dennis and I didn't have the privilege of growing old together, they're only half right: Dennis *did* grow old with me. I just didn't grow old with him.

This is the first day where tensions between allopathic medicine and palliative care engage in combat and lock around Dennis's care. It happens often but not always.

There are scenes for us here that would make lovely commercials for palliative medicine. I cling to these for my life—for my Dennis's life—but I am keenly aware of a dangerous anxiety threatening my ability to think clearly. I page my psychiatrist, Dr. Anna, as much because I cannot be clear about my anxiety as because I feel it overwhelming me. She is gracious and reassuring in ways that make me believe that I can do what these days implicitly require of me. Everyone should have a Dr. Anna.

A couple of days ago, I could extract a breathy, labored "I love you" from Dennis simply by announcing the obvious: "I love you, Dream Man." The fact that this was clearly reflexive did not detract from its sweet sound. In some ways I loved it even more for just that fact. It was coerced, but it was comforting. My husband no longer spoke volitionally, but he loved me reflexively. Now there is a period of roughly twenty-four hours when I hear only lonely words, separate and distinct in time and context from others: "sorry," "ten," "up," "can't." Dennis's eyes are closed as he pushes his head back deeper into his pillow. And somewhere between the reflexive love and the last random words is my husband's last sentence: "The car needs washing." Sometimes the truth is not romantic.

Brittany seems to have a good sense of how words fit at the end of someone's life. She has been in close phone contact during this hospitalization but has not seen either of her parents since we have settled into crisis mode. Her last image of her Dad came watching his back and mine moving purposefully and laboriously to the southbound train that would deposit us in the City to begin yet another of the usual sorts of hospitalization. Or so we anticipated at that time. That was a week ago. Brittany traveled out of state to be with friends and planned another trip two days later in the other direction. "I think maybe I'll come to visit Dad tomorrow sometime. What do you think?" she asks.

"You know I trust your judgment and that I will be supportive of whatever you decide. But...Britt? I need you to understand something clearly."

"Yeah...?" She sounds braced and frightened. I wish I could hold her right now to shore her up and myself in the process, but I am not leaving my husband in the hospital, and she's afraid to see her dad here. So we're doing some tough talking through cell lines. I can hear her heartbeat, and I can see the emotional fence she's hiding behind in some vain hope that not acknowledging reality will somehow change it.

"I can't promise you that there will always be a tomorrow. I think you're really asking me if you have my blessing not to come at all." I steel myself for her rebuttal, but it doesn't come.

"Yeah, I guess I am...I just don't think that my relationship with Dad can be measured by how long I sit beside him in a hospital when he doesn't even know I am there." She sounds defensive.

"No, this is just the good-bye part. You have twenty-two years of being Daddy's girl. All the ways that he invested in you and all the experiences you shared? None of those will go away. If you don't want another hospital scene, that's okay. But it's important to me that the decision is yours. *I* don't want to be blamed if you make a choice that you later regret."

She doesn't say a word, but as her mother, I can hear something akin to, "I can't believe we are having this conversation," in her silence. Nor can I.

"Why don't you just go to Dad's closet and put on one of his sweaters? I'll talk to you tomorrow." She sniffles. I pray out loud with her. We hang up. I imagine her burying her face in one of her dad's favorite sweaters and sobbing because Dennis's solid presence does not wrap his arms around her and hold her to his chest. I cry with her.

Roughly four minutes later, I get another call from Brittany's cell phone: "Okay, so I am heading south on Route 41. What exit do I take?" There is no reference that might lead the casual observer to suspect that we had just had any exchange at all and certainly not a candid exchange about what this twenty-two-year-old girl's last time with her dad will look like. Much as we both want to build more memories of life, the only one available to us is one of death. I look at the clock. Our girls keep different hours than we do. It will be close to 11:00 p.m. before Brittany arrives at the hospital. I get the razor from his shaving kit and prepare to give Dennis a bit of tidying up for his last visit with his firstborn daughter. I have removed his hospital gown because it was wet with his perspiration and tangled with his thrashing and my repositioning of him. I put a clean one on. I straighten the bedding. I go through my mouth care routine: the comer of a damp wash cloth along the inside of his cheeks, another comer around his lips, toothpaste on my finger so as not to irritate his fragile gums, a final comer of a wash cloth with clean water to rid his mouth of the paste that would otherwise collect where his lips might hinge if he could smile. Then he gets a cursory pass of the deodorant he always uses. I do everything I can to make this dying man look like our daughter's father. I finish just as her diminutive frame appears in the doorway.

She stands rigid and frightened, willing her round, blue-green eyes not to cry. That child came home from the hospital on her dad's thirtieth birthday over twenty-two years ago. Now she is in another one in another part of the country to say good-bye to him. Britt has a baseball cap pulled low over her long, blond curls. Dennis loves those curls. Dennis loves this girl. She waits for me to hug her and draw her into the space she instinctively knows is holy ground. She stands a couple of feet from the end of his bed. He's not moving, and his eyes are closed. She's not moving, and her eyes are fixed on him. "Does Dad know I am here?" she whispers.

"Hearing is the last sense to leave a person. I think he knows we're with him, and that will bring him a measure of peace. But he won't be able to speak back, and we won't know for sure what he hears. He's very weak."

"Then it would be really annoying if I talk to him," she reasons. "I should just sing." For about twenty minutes, Brittany weaves through songs that her dad taught her, popular hits they both enjoyed, and a few from her dad's favorite artist, Bruce Springsteen. When she starts to sing Nat King Cole's "Unforgettable," she stops after a couple of bars to look at me sheepishly and reveal: "Dad and I were going to record this for you as a duet but we never did…" I resist the urge to be disappointed and focus on how privileged I am that bits of Dennis's music are embodied in his girl.

"I get to hear it now," I assure her. She sings with a haunting intensity and easily fills the space between them that earlier seemed so achingly empty. When she's done with her concert, she stands abruptly and kisses her dad on the cheek. At the elevators, she gives me a quick hug, turns first away and then back for a tighter version of that hug, and says softly, "I guess I should *really* hug the people I can."

TALKING POINTS FOR MORTALS

1. In what ways might you benefit from changing the focus of your treatment from curative to comfort care?

2. In what ways is such a concept threatening to you and/or to those who love you?

■ ■ ■

CHAPTER 9

Allopathy

[uh-lop-uh-thee] n. system of medicine which opposes or suppresses disease by using antithetical interventions; conventional western medicine

This day has an auspicious beginning. It is Monday, and the hospital is at full staff again. I'm pleased that Dr. Ali rather than a new face is heading the palliative team. Perhaps best of all, Dr. Anna has offered to visit before her otherwise full day begins. I know that she has to take a very early train to make this happen. She also needs an umbrella on this particular morning. I suppose she needs coffee, too, but I have none to offer. She is surprised to find us in a different room than I had given the day before. Dennis had been moved to a designated isolation room because of the possibility of shingles having appeared as sores on his hip and thigh. When I apologize, she counters quickly, "It's just my anxiety around what's happening." There is plenty of that going around.

Something about having an MD I deeply respect express her personal anxiety around our situation ministers profoundly to some raw place in me. I check quickly to be sure that Dennis does not need me, and we slip past the double doors and down the hall to a private conference space. We sit side by side on the little sofa. A highly professional woman, Dr. Anna turns quickly to assess how I'm holding up. She studies me. I am grateful for her attention. I realize that I am more peaceful than the circumstances would predict and I tell her how precious these days are to me. I do not hold the words that pass between us as much as the balm of being heard and understood. Dr. Anna practices medicine in this large hospital and moves easily through the system of discrete specialties and functions. At the same time, though, she is able to see beyond her official roles to the patient systems impacted by her practice. It is a sacrificial way to care for patients, and I am grateful. When I escort her to the elevators and turn back to my charge, I am in a better place to greet the challenges of the day. And there will be many.

We have been running an end game around Dr. Stefanowicz on the assumption that if she had anything in her bag of tricks they would have been used already. The purpose of the contact now is to obtain a consultation from the MD who has known Dennis during the full three-year diagnosed course of his disease. It is a clinically wise and professionally courteous gesture. I have no evidence that Dr. Stefanowicz understands the devastation her carefully catalogued symptoms and deficits are wreaking in Dennis's life. I do not deliberately keep her to of the loop; I simply see no reason to include her. Dr. Jamie consults Dennis's specialist of record, Dr. Stefanowicz, as a matter of course. We are living at the hospital under the care of the palliative service. This is likely the end of Dennis's life, and I want to be as proactive as I can be in advocating for his dying well. Until the very end of his life, I wake each day believing that this is a reasonable and feasible goal.

I'm surprised when Dr. Stefanowicz arrives in Dennis's room. At first I do not recognize her, garbed in the yellow protective gear required when a patient is under isolation precautions. In this case, these precautions were lifted after skin sores were deemed to be coma sores and not shingles, but the supply cart is still outside the room and the MD is being cautious. The large, loose yellow gown coupled with the face mask fitted around her blond head makes her look like the Michelin man after a bath in some yellow paint. She does not smile as she enters the room. I don't either, for which I feel some guilt. I want to be a bigger person than that. I know I must be exuding the discomfort I feel as Dr. Stefanowicz begins her examination. "Do you know who I am?" she asks him repeatedly. "Do you recognize me?" He does not respond verbally, but he does open his eyes for a moment.

"I think the mask makes it hard for him to see you," I offer.

"Dennis, squeeze my hand." I cannot tell if he does or not, but he has been roused from his stupor by the cadence and pressure of her speech. "Dennis, stick out your tongue." This he does. The whole encounter seems bizarre. Dr. Stefanowicz is attempting to do an examination on a person who is not verbalizing more than single words strewn at increasingly disparate intervals throughout the day. His eyes are almost always closed. The only response he seems to evidence is the perpetual grimace. A knock on the door draws me out to greet the attorney who had been completing the process of putting Dennis's affairs in order prior to this hospitalization. We speak for a few minutes outside Dennis's room before Dr. Stefanowicz emerges.

"He did recognize me after a while," she offers as she begins to extricate herself from the yellow Michelin costume. Then she looks at me with the flattest of flat affects and says quite surely, "I have never seen this before. It is *not* progression of the diagnosed disease." Her recommendation is a full workup to determine what is happening medically. I have already given this option quite a bit of thought, and I don't hesitate in responding to her.

"Even if there were some other disease process on top of the current known diagnosis, Dennis would still be trapped in this body with extraordinary and unremitting pain. I would not treat an anomaly and effectively prolong his suffering."

"Well, this is not the diagnosed disease." She is as clear about her perspective as I am about mine. She leaves, and I realize suddenly that my heart is racing and my breathing is fast and shallow. I take a few deep breaths, look at my husband lying still in the big bed with its mechanical turning and inflating, and seethe in sync with it.

A crystalline chill goes through me as my legal business is completed, and I pull a chair up to Dennis's bed and sling my legs over one arm and twist to rest my cheek near his. Dr. Stefanowicz is saying that Dennis's known disease process could not be causing what I think of as end-of-life symptoms: wild fluctuation in his respiration, periods of apnea lasting as long as thirty seconds, peripheral edema, anorexia, wasting, and lack of communication. Without an end-of-life diagnosis, however, protocol would preclude the palliative team from offering all the care that would otherwise be available. For a nanosecond I consider the full body workup just to prove what I knew intuitively: that there is no additional disease beyond the one that I have watched segment by linear segment in some sort of frightening geometric arc.

A full week after this hospitalization started, Dennis's pain is not effectively managed. He has developed bedsores in part because his body is shutting down but also because even the most careful repositioning causes him so obvious and horrifying discomfort that hospital staff shies from the task unless I ask them to help me with it. A full workup would require Dennis to be off the special bed that undulates beneath him. It would separate me for hours from this man I do not trust to the system. I know that these hours tumbling one on the other are a precious bridge to a time that I think of as the "rest of my life." I elect to wait and see what happens. The dramatic tension is building on the stage of our lives. Dennis is dying. Of this I am sure. Much as I would dearly like to extend his life, I will not prolong the process of dying. The machines known as "hospital protocol" and the "US health care system" unfortunately seem to be winding up as we are winding down.

Dr. Sue Jacks is a pain specialist whom we met during Dennis's initial admission assessment. She's not only an integral part of the palliative team, but to my mind, she is the person most likely to be able to mitigate if not eradicate Dennis's complex pain syndrome. From the start, her clipped speech and narrow-eyed intensity impressed me. She is analytical and precise by temperament. She brings this style with her into Dennis's room on one of these last days. Dr. Jacks does not mince words.

Nurse Jane is equally thoughtful. Her gentle manner is evidenced both in what she says (not much) and how she says it (quietly). Like Dr. Jacks, Jane considers words an economic good to be appropriated conservatively. Somehow, I never think I know what she is thinking, but I nonetheless believe that she cares deeply. As the days run into each other, both professionals speak less often. This is good. Their weighted words come at the vulnerable places I try to guard. On this day, they come to Dennis's room late in the afternoon. They are carrying paperwork held up to their chests like armor. It strikes me, at the time, that these women have shields. I, on the other hand, do not. I'm at that particular moment kneeling on the head of Dennis's bed to the left of his pillow. My arms are tucked around his shoulder, and my head rests close enough to feel his breath on my cheek. After a quick greeting, Dr. Jacks frowns thoughtfully and bends over to meet my eyes: "Who is the physician that knows Dennis the best? Who is the one who has known him the longest?" I can see where this is going.

"That's not the same person!" I hear the edge in my voice, and it surprises me. I don't want to be rude. I think of other professionals beyond the one specialist he met at the time of his initial diagnosis. Perhaps the palliative care MD who continued to make house calls even after Dennis was discharged from another hospice for extended prognosis last year? Perhaps the sympathetic pain specialist who also practices at another city hospital? Anyhow, this thinking has no place right now. I am busy with my charge as Dennis's functional companion. Dennis moans, and I speak to him, holding his head and fabricating reassuring utterances to soothe him: "I know, Dream. The medical team is working to come up with a way for you to get comfortable. I'm right here. I won't leave you. I'm right here." I cradle his cheek and put my hand across his increasingly rutted brow as if love alone can soothe his pain.

"Can we step out of the room?" This request from Dr. Jacks is reasonable. To insulate a patient from some of the anxiety of the care team is wise. It does strike me that Dennis and I are so much in the habit of functioning as a unit. Now in a perverse reversal as the stakes are mounting, I am alone to represent us both. I unfurl myself from my awkward contortion on Dennis's bed and follow the two women out of the room. Like I said, I know where this is going.

"Dr. Stefanowicz does not believe that Dennis is experiencing simple disease progression. She has recommended a full workup...It is highly likely that Dennis will live for many months longer. We will need to begin discussing a discharge plan for him."

"I believe that Dennis is actively dying and that some of the behaviors noted today are terminal agitation. Other people might lash out in pain or frustration, but not

Dennis...and certainly not Dennis to *me*." This is my conviction, and I suspect I will need to repeat it quite a few times in advocating for end-of-life care. Jane looks down as if she would like to sink into the floor, but it doesn't yield.

"Dennis will come home if he doesn't meet the criteria to stay here through the end of his life." Now I'm looking at the same spot of floor as Jane. It doesn't yield to me either. I want to scream something, and I am sensing that the battle to stave off tears can go on only so long before I crumble. I look back through the glass door at my disintegrating husband. "How is his pain going to be controlled at home if it cannot be managed here?"

I'm angry and I'm frightened and I'm not sure how to best advocate for Dennis. Should I just bring him home with hospice support and rid myself of these battles? Or should I keep lobbying for Dennis to be allowed palliative sedation until his body slips into a different place—a place without pain?

> I can only imagine how you, Other Wife, will come to terms with what you are experiencing. Again I pray for you to have the wisdom and grace to endure these days. I know some of your fears, and I share your anxieties. How much easier this would be if we could collaborate in the middle of all of this. I would love to get some ideas from you.

"Hospices have different guidelines for the use of medications..." Dr. Jacks drones. I know this. It's my profession. I also know that Dennis well meets criteria for hospice admission. This is determined by a specific list of symptoms for each diagnosis and concludes with the sentence, "With usual disease progression life expectancy is less than six months."

Palliative medicine frightens people because of its association with death. I understand that apprehension, but for me, palliation offers a hope around death that is otherwise absent. It is a philosophical approach to care that attends to distressing symptoms while acknowledging that death is approaching. Once death is accepted as inevitable—and of course it is for all of us at some point—patients and loved ones can lean into it rather than waste increasingly precious energy railing against it

It's a losing battle, Other Wife. You don't want to get caught in it.

Not able to think of anything both honest and edifying, I just stand for some fraction of a minute considering my options in silence. Without another utterance from any of us, I turn back to the mechanicals of mutual soothing in which Dennis and I now indulge ourselves while the horrifying realities of what is to come preclude my doing much else. I worry that I am rude.

It's important not to alienate the professionals on whom your dear one's care is dependent. I'm sure that you know that, Other Wife. Maybe you're doing a better job than I am right now. But I know there's no one else on this earth more committed to Dennis

than I am. With that commitment comes a commensurate amount of responsibility. I feel the battle for end-of-life peace for Dennis raging not only in his body but throughout this hospital. There are interactions like the one described here that cause me considerable anxiety—as if I don't already have enough of that.

I try not to cry. I'm successful, but all those unshed tears gather within me. They seize the muscles of my back, oscillate in my head, and pool in my chest. I try not to be overwhelmed with the practical demands of this day. I try not to think. "Enjoy his presence. Enjoy his presence. Enjoy…" I tell myself over and over until the flood of my own body and soul recedes. I'm sure of only two things right now: Dennis is dying, and any moments I lose with him I will never be able to return and gather. He moans quietly, having exhausted his capacity even to suffer with any gusto. His flushed, flaccid form challenges me to find my Dennis, and I accept the challenge as I rearrange my body around his bed and settle into that physical space where we are still a couple.

As I set my mind on the ethics of my Dennis's care, Dr. Kara stops to see us. She folds her compact frame into a chair near the head of Dennis's bed while her eyes take in the scene: another illustration of how to drape myself around the hospital furniture, and the soft brushing of his thinned and graying hair with my fingers. Her generous nature fills the space. She has a manner that seems to magnify whatever good can be found in a situation. "I love coming in here. I wish other families could see this,"

Dr. Kara says. I'm not sure what she means. But I need any affirmation I can get.

"Dennis deserves whatever love I can pour over him." I point to the eight-and-a-half-by-eleven sheet of paper with its boldly marked statistical outlier to the right of the bell curve and its tail. "That's the visual description of the man in this bed." I'm reminded of the fight that led me to want to be so clear in communicating my in-spite-of-it-all commitment. I am reminded of how complicated life can be. Dr. Kara shares the quiet, private space with us for a while. We talk about the place of palliative medicine in the US health care system. We talk about our kids. We talk about what life is going to be like when this vigil ends and my life without Dennis begins. By this time, Dr. Kara has earned my full respect, and she uses it as leverage to encourage me to seek bereavement services for myself and my daughters. As she heads for the door, she pauses to tell me that there is an ethics committee meeting scheduled for the next morning and that I should expect a call from Dr. Maggie Gallagher about meeting privately with her.

"I'm nervous," I admit. Dr. Kara studies me for a moment and then she shakes her head slowly as her eyes bore into mine.

"Just tell her the truth," she advises simply, hugs me, and leaves. I spend the rest of the evening and much of the night praying that my thinking would be linear and that my truth would resonate with these key decision makers.

Fast-forward a few weeks: 730 pages of official medical records from Dennis's last hospitalization are in a stack on the table. I expect to surrender a week or two to reading and augmenting my understanding of those last days of Dennis's life. But it takes less than two hours. And to file it in chronological order—which for some strange reason is not how medical records print. The medication administration record—known within the health care system as the MAR—was meticulously documented. Drug names, concentrations, dosing and titration rates, times bags were hung on the IV pole or inserted into so-called "smart pumps" (which are not very smart) are all recorded. But only a pharmacist might (possibly) believe that my husband's MAR told a story. It does outline a course of care riddled with treatment failure and care plan changes and increasingly, desperately high doses of medication. But it tells nothing of the drama of end-of-life care. It tells nothing of Dennis as unique in the entire world. Most MD visits were not even noted, let alone used to document the intense interactions in Dennis's room and in meeting rooms throughout the hospital during the course of his admission. RN documentation excluded interactions with Dennis and with me and in one case even with one of our daughters on the phone as she struggled to understand how ill her dad really was. Yet without exception, these skilled caregivers interacted routinely and compassionately. In some cases they did so with tears in their eyes.

To acknowledge humanity is to admit a profound complexity at end of life. Recorded or not, the winding down of a life is emotionally intense for the medical community as well as for loved ones. And it should be. From the first day of medical school, MDs have been focused on saving life. Their considerable intellect, formal training, and clinical experience turn to a symptom—a discrete physical problem. This is the allopathic model on which the US medial system is based. People are construed as a conglomeration of isolatable cells, organs, and physical systems. MDs are assigned their piece of that puzzle. But the truth is that most MDs seem puzzled much of the time.

It's not only the US health care system that sees Dennis as the composite of various parts. On occasion, as Dennis's disease progresses, I find myself seeing him from the dispassionate stance of an anthropologist. I've watched a man age thirty years in the span of less than three. Sometimes when I come upon him from behind, I find myself taking an allopathic inventory of this man. Without the watery blue eyes or dimples (the left is deeper than the right, as is true of each of Janet Purcell Sheehan's seven children) or the face of the man looking at me, I more easily separate my husband from what I observe. From the back, I can see the increasingly fine hair with more and more silver overtaking the dark brown base. Dennis's hairline has changed because it seems like the flesh of his face is being pulled to somewhere deep within him to feed the disease. The back of his neck has a crease running parallel to his shoulders that I only recently notice. This man—all Dennis but not at all him—does not stand erect and strong with chest thrust forward into the next adventure. He stoops not only by rounding his shoulders but also by giving way around his middle, where he has barely enough muscle to be upright at all. The resultant, curved profile is not symmetrical. His left side is stronger, which torques his torso slightly clockwise. This man's gait is labored and unsteady. The emaciated legs hanging from his trunk do not dangle the loose flesh I would have anticipated with such rapid wasting. Instead, the flesh seems to be pulled tight into his body somewhere, as if in a desperate attempt to anchor his limbs. Dennis falls routinely, and typically hard. He always gets up. One lump on his head troubled him for weeks. An unfortunate intersection of scapula and floor never did heal, in spite of time and physical therapy.

Then the man turns, and for a fraction of a moment I see my Dennis. I see the pale-blue ocean eyes, which he would say are his best feature. I see those dimples. I see the ruddy Irish coloring. Overlaying this familiar facial topography, I also see an alien landscape: blotchy, fever-skinned, and deeply furrowed. The terrain on the bridge of his nose is especially rugged. I hear as well as see the open-mouthed breathing, which emanates louder as the fatigue of the day encroaches on him. I'm losing my very wonderful husband, and in his place is a very sick, old man.

Many weeks later, when I read Dennis's autopsy report, I see again how the health care system reduces people to their parts. It began with a paragraph of prose, not all of which was accurate. It stated the obvious—but until that time officially unacknowledged—"looks older than his reported fifty-two years." Individual organs were listed in capital letters and underlined. After most of these followed the observation, "Unremarkable." All I could think was that *none* of it was unremarkable to me. Relationship is what makes the man: the relationships of physical parts to one another, the relationships of his physical system to his psychosocial reality, and, from my perspective the most important of all, the relationship of my Dennis to me and to the rest of his family and social circle. A man is not, as it turns out, the sum of his parts. As Dennis got sicker and his death more and more inevitable, he put his hand on my shoulder, fixed his eyes on mine, and said slowly, "No matter what happens, I will never be far from you because my handprint is so deep in your heart." I wonder, when the time comes for my autopsy, if the pathologist will find that handprint.

TALKING POINTS FOR MORTALS

1. What specialists are involved in your care?
2. How might their services be better coordinated?
3. Who is your "quarterback," both among your loved ones and your medical team?

■ ■ ■

CHAPTER 10

Ethics

[eth-iks] n. framework within which moral philosophy informs code of behavior in an attempt to arrive at right conduct

The message I e-mailed to our family and friends that afternoon read as follows:

Well, the BIG meeting with the Smart People took four hours, and they have decided on a new drug mix to sedate Dennis. As of early afternoon it is working. I am SO grateful. Because of the medical goals (sedation) and the personal realities (Dennis can't visit and I want to focus on him), we continue to ask you to channel all that enormous desire to DO something into a "bank" for later. We will have needs I can only begin to imagine...and I am pretty creative.

I'm still creative. I still depend heavily on the sense that our girls and I are living, in Dennis's wake, with a remarkable support system.

Ever since I met you, dear Other Wife, lying on the floor of the ICU, you have shadowed me from the inside. I thought about you in the middle of interactions with the palliative team, and I know that they would be of such comfort to you. I imagined you navigating the machines known as the hospital or the US health care system or insurance, and I could touch your anxiety. I willed you to keep asking questions and to speak what was in your heart… and never to lose visceral contact with your dear one in hat bed.

The Other Wife keeps me company through the long nights and weary days in the hospital. But never is she more viscerally present than the day of the ethics committee meeting. I am keenly aware that, even as I speak to my husband's care, I also serve as her advocate. And I am as much committed to her case as I am to my own.

> *I picture you, Other Wife, a week into the brutal routine of work and hospital and household. You're exhausted. You're increasingly frightened at the apparent lack of improvement in your husband's condition. Last night there was a message left on your home phone by a doctor asking for a meeting with you. You don't recognize the name or the voice, but you get a little time off to be at the hospital at the appointed time. The doctor takes you to a little conference room and gently asks questions about your husband's care. You do your best to focus on each question, but you don't have many answers. And the ones about what sort of care your husband wants at the end of life? You never talked about any of that.*

But for me? Well, Dennis and I have talked about end-of-life care a great deal. We talked about it sideways because of my work as a medical social worker. I forced Dennis to review every sad scenario I encountered in a (vain) attempt to protect us both from being in a place where dying well would be impossible. We talked about our own preferences head-on because of my complicated medical history and because Dennis had a nasty form of an uncontrolled progressive illness. I'm not in the same place as that Other Wife. When I have my audience with the chair of the ethics committee, I'm fixed on my job as Dennis's medical quarterback and the guardian of his end-of-life experience. As I spill our story, Dr. Gallagher listens gently, leaning in. At the end of our conversation, she asks gingerly if I would be willing to speak to the full ethics committee, which is gathering in another room. Specifically, she says, "I think the committee would benefit if they could hear you tell them your story."

Envisioning a group of four or five members of the medical team, I don't flinch in agreeing.

"I would consider that a privilege," I say politely.

An hour later, this same efficiently gracious MD escorts me to another conference room. The door opens to a room with an expansive table framed two deep by professionals numbering perhaps twenty-five or more. A seat at the head of the table is empty, but I regain enough composure to make some joke about the size of my audience and slide into a chair that feels somehow less prominent. It is only a token gesture; wherever I sit will functionally be the center of this room.

While the professionals in the room—MDs, PhDs, RNs, and ancillary staff—listen, Dr. Gallagher asks me to share what I told her. I had thought that all the big decisions were made and the patient and family wishes made clear by conversation and written documentation of the Health Care Power of Attorney. Looking at all these people gathered, I'm flattened by the sense that I will not be able to successfully advocate for what I perceive as a good death—having enough medication to mitigate Dennis's unremitting pain and, perhaps as compelling to me, the existential suffering that accompanies it. My dismay serves me well. Calculating the odds, I have no reason to be cautious. Still, I mentally scroll through my strategy: tell the truth, tell the story, and stay linear. It is a strategy boiled down from the direct counsel of Dr. Kara and Dr. Maggie and from my own awareness of MDs as scientists.

With a deep breath, I begin. "If I were an MD or a PhD at a major US teaching hospital and a group of specialists said one thing and the wife said another, I would go with the specialists. But in this case, I think that would be a mistake." I describe Dennis's unusual medical condition with as much data as I have to buttress my assertions. I'm observant, medically trained, and committed with every fiber of my being to advocating for this man to whom I vowed before the God of the universe to love in sickness as well as in health. Health seems such a distant memory. No, not even a memory, but a barely discernible fairy tale that I once enjoyed.

The ethics committee is meeting to determine two elements of Dennis's situation. The first is whether the symptoms that could be construed as end of life are caused by disease progression, as I contend, or rather by the aggressive attempts to treat his intractable pain in recent days. The second issue is whether the symptoms could ethically be treated, knowing that Dennis's life might be shortened by their administration. There is, in fact, a legal safeguard for MDs with this concern. The doctrine of double effect acknowledges that there are some highly valuable interventions at end of life, which are known to also compromise vital system functions. In Dennis's case, the main issue is that the medications that might ease his suffering will also compromise his breathing and ability to protect his airway. It is this same law that Dr. Kara invoked while interacting with Dr. Bjorn on the ICU when we were resisting Dennis's being a full code. It is this law that provides some hope that Dennis might be freed of his suffering.

I'm asked, "What would you like to have happen?"

I choke on my answer. I stutter: "What do I *want*? What I *want* is for Dennis to get miraculously better and celebrate our twenty-fifth wedding anniversary with me in September, but I understand that I cannot have what I want."

Dr. Jacks asks, "What do you see happening here?"

I fight the urge to scream that I am a wife mired in anticipatory grief who has been sleeping in a hospital chair for a week at this point. I adore my husband enough to call him Dream Man, and I am watching him die. I want to remind these brilliant people that they are the ones who are supposed to be fielding the questions. I elect to feign calmness and continue on my planned trajectory: tell the truth, tell the story, and stay linear.

"I think Dennis is actively dying based on his edema, apnea, decubiti ulcers, and the congestion that I hear and suspect is an aspiration pneumonia. That suggests that he will only be alive another few days regardless of treatment." I take a breath and pan the room. Who is with me, I wonder? Who finds it irritating or even offensive that I am speaking like a peer in this room where people have lots of important letters trailing their names? I regroup by playing my mantra: tell the truth, tell the story, and stay linear.

"I could bring him home with hospice support where, undermedicated, he will likely need to be physically restrained by me, with our daughters bearing witness. I would hate for these girls to see me fighting their dad as he dies in front of them. I would hate to risk their seeing me as their dad's adversary, when for their whole lives they have had the privilege of knowing that we were committed to one another above all else. Alternatively, if this committee allows it, Dennis could remain here at the hospital with enough medication to ease his suffering. That would be my preference." Dr. Gallagher notes references to our faith in the medical record.

"Can you please clarify the implications of your faith this for the committee?"

I'm not sure what to say, so I go back to my game plan: tell the truth, tell the story, and stay linear.

"Dennis and I have a strong conviction that God is sovereign. Because of this conviction, he has been able to be remarkably brave in spite of excruciating and unremitting pain over the past three years. Sometimes he presents as less dramatically ill because of his faith." The room is quiet. I wait for the next question. It appears that I have an audience, and I break from linear just a bit in order to tell the truth and tell the story. I am grateful that these professionals have all taken time from their days to discuss Dennis's care plan. I introduce them to the Other Wife. I do not think that she would know how to take advantage of the privilege of such a meeting should she ever find herself in one. I ask the ethics committee to consider her, too, as they wade through data and sort through emotions and verify protocol in this day when Dennis is the identified patient. I worry that perhaps I should not have broadened the lens of this committee, but the Other Wife has been with me throughout this grim season. I'm committed to helping her in this war even if I lose my own battle.

Jennifer, the nurse who has been with Dennis for the majority of his twelve-hour days, speaks to her observations of my devotion to Dennis. "I just want to say that Susan has been so attentive to Dennis…When I am dying, I would love to have her with me…She never loses it in front of him."

Well, of course, I *have* lost all of it as my heart bounces around in my chest cavity and my tears stagnate somewhere in my throat. But the sentiment is sweet, and I'm grateful not to be demonized. I'm aware that there are some in the room who believe that I came to the hospital effectively to secure physician-assisted suicide. That is not a legal option in Illinois, nor is it my desire. What I am requesting is so personally simple and yet medically complex. I want some relief, or in my wildest dreams, even mitigation of pain as Dennis dies.

Again I wait in the silence of this crowd for another question. Many are unspoken. They hang heavy and never find audible words. I cannot resist a tease: "Now you guys have nothing to say?" Thankfully the room lightens a bit.

An MD looks from the hands folded in his lap to my face and then quickly away. "I can only imagine what you and your husband have been through. You have my prayers." His compassion is obvious.

"Yours and half of the western hemisphere," I note. "I can be strong here because there is an army out there praying with us." And with that I am excused while the ethics committee continues to confer.

As I leave the room I'm fairly confident we have lost. The bottom line is that my testimony differs from that of a group of specialists. But as hours pass by without news, the more grueling the wait, the higher I think my odds of a win. Surely if there were no chance at all, these many professionals would have gone back to their day jobs. Maybe they forgot to tell me? Maybe no one volunteered to bring such grim news? I'm aware of the head game volleying in my brain. I will myself to attend to Dennis and to step out of the ethics game until I have facts to work with.

Our youngest daughter, Juliana, anticipating her twenty-first birthday at the time, provides me some diversion. Juliana has come to the hospital to see her dad for the second time. She knows that it will be emotionally difficult, and she arrives with three of her friends who are content to wait in a sitting room. They offer to "do anything" for me. One goes off to find some food. Another accepts the mission of finding a charger for my cell phone. After I spend some time with them as a group, I escort Juliana to her dad's room. I can't help but be so proud of this girl with her dad's dimples and Irish complexion and watery blue eyes. I can't help but be grateful for her presence. After Juliana and her friends leave the city, I move the hospital-issue, avocado-green Naugahyde recliner perpendicular to Dennis's bed. I lie on my belly and rest my upper body in the curve at Dennis's waist. He has not eaten in week, and his five-ten frame likely weighs less than 140 pounds. His left hip protrudes.

At some point in the early afternoon, I see members of the ethics committee in the corridors. One does not make eye contact with me; that must be a bad sign. One of them appears not to see me at all, which I register as neutral. Dr. Gallagher is moving at a clip more like speed walking than anything else. She tells me quite simply that the committee has determined that Dennis can be given palliative sedation, but there is some protocol that needs to be addressed in order to administer this medication on the palliative floor. For a moment I am elated. We won!

Then I remember that my husband is dying and I feel ill. To lobby with everything in me for the loss of what I want most in this world to hold requires the suspension of parts of myself. I again wonder how the Other Wife will steer through this crazy-making maze. I am okay to do this without someone at my elbow. I wonder who will come alongside the Other Wife as my professional experience steers me. Over the next few hours, a new drug—the last opiate in the arsenal—is started to tide Dennis over until an exception to hospital protocol will allow the initiation of palliative sedation. For about thirty minutes, it seems to scramble Dennis's central nervous system, and he rests comfortably. After that, the dose is ratcheted up periodically. Dennis's rest is still fitful, but there are moments when he does not moan. And there are moments when he is sedated deeply enough that I can press my head into that warm spot between his clavicle and his ear without bothering him. I doze there for a bit and wake to the realization that we have not had the privilege of sleeping this close for months.

By nine thirty that night, I have changed into Dennis's boxers and one of the T-shirts I had packed for my husband's hospital stay but that became impractical as he became sicker and sicker and the mechanics of getting anything more than a sheet over him became too difficult. Wearing his clothes is one way I find to get close to my husband even as he slips further from me.

The change of shift comes, and I spend some time with the night nurse getting to know her a bit and making sure that she knows my husband. Dennis is calm and not moving too much, so I steal a moment to e-mail friends. When I return to the room, I see Dr. Gallagher. She is still fully engaged in the business of unraveling and rewinding Dennis's care. She has a pile of documentation in her arms. I am sure she is exhausted, but she is warm, and I am grateful. I sleep more that night than on any other in this room to which my life is now limited.

TALKING POINTS FOR MORTALS

1. What are your highest values?
2. How do these values interface with your medical situation?
3. Are these values consistent with the standards that your loved ones affirm?
4. Are these values consistent with the standards that you medical team exhibits around your treatment?

■ ■ ■

CHAPTER 11

Sentinel

[sen-tn-1] n. guard watching for unexpected and critical threats to integrity of others

I n hospital parlance, a sentinel event is one for which the hospital accreditation board demands a report and, subsequently, a root-cause analysis. It is a complicated and arduous process. While such analysis puts staff on the defensive, it can also be very useful in improving future performance. As Dennis's case becomes more and more controversial, I'm keenly aware that every step we take will affect future protocols, just as those who have gone before us were impacting us. I fight for Dennis's best interest with every ounce of my being and, for the sake of the Other Wife, lobby for the betterment of the system.

> *I've e-mailed my friends and family the same things I would like to tell you, Other Wife. I'm thinking about your friends and families too. I imagine everyone who*

cares about you is going about their days somewhat distracted by your situation. I figure it's in our best interest to keep them informed en masse. A "dear friends and family" e-mail will save you a lot of redundant conversations. I know that you would like each loved one to feel that they're given your personal attention, and I know that they covet that from you, but this is the time in life to suspend social convention and conserve as much energy as you possibly can. This is what I wrote on day nine of Dennis's hospital stay:

"The Smart People are still conferring. It is now clear that Dennis is a statistical outlier. I TOLD them that already, and I know that each of you taking the time to read this would concur! His medical situation is so complex that it has become a lightning rod for the Smart People. In some weird sense this makes the emotional toll easier for me. Health care advocacy is hard work. Please continue to pray for the palliative service. They are a remarkable group of people working very, very hard to allow Dennis some sustained comfort. No, we're not there yet, but we're getting closer. And yes, I really am fine here. Go figure. I won't be later, but now my job is clear and where there is clarity I am happiest. For my Britt and Juliana, this is less fine. They are both doing a good job taking care of themselves and each other..."

My personal sentinel, Dr. Anna, makes a second dawn visit today. Her face in the door's window reveals the gracious intensity I think of as her hallmark. She is purpose-ful. She is compassionate. To have these attributes trained on me by a more than competent psychiatrist is a privilege, and so I extract as much as I can from our time together on the little sofa in the hospice family room. Someone has left the flat-screen TV on. Fumbling with the remote, I can't figure out how to eliminate its incessant demand for our attention. Dr. Anna easily makes it stop. Similarly, she quiets the distractions pulling at my deeper sensibilities. I tell her of some the conversations the day before at the ethics committee meeting and around Dennis's bed. She listens intently as if to a good piece of fiction. But she understands that this is my life, and her eyes widen. "You really said that?"

"Well, yes. Yes. I did."

The thrill of being heard against all odds mounts anew from somewhere deep within me. In the moment, I pur-pose to keep saying whatever I need to say for Dennis and for the Other Wife. I will fill the role as Dennis's advocate with all that my forty-seven-year-old self has developed to be. I will bring the whole package to bear to advocate for the best possible death Dennis's bizarre physical reality will allow. I will press the Allopathic team to see Dennis as the remarkable warrior that he is. I will honor him by advocat-ing to the best of my ability until he takes his last arduous breath. In all of this, I will not forget my friend the Other Wife.

As I understand it this morning, the considered opinion of the ethics committee is that Dennis is deemed eligible for palliative sedation in light of the extreme realities of dis-ease progression in general and of his excruciating pain in particular. But, as far as I know, the administrative sign-off to go ahead with Dennis's new drug cocktail has still not come in. I'm holding out for the Propofol, a quick-acting anesthetic that I think is Dennis's best chance of pain relief. I expect the bureaucratic machine to grind out their exception first thing this morning. I'm up early and waiting eagerly. I hope I appear to be waiting patiently, although in fact I am not. Dennis is assigned a new RN that day who doesn't know him. Marla, clearly a capable professional, bustles warmly around Dennis. She does what needs to be done with efficiency and gentleness. I'm grateful she's also willing to limit her poking and prodding, her measurements of what amounts to the pace of Dennis's death, in deference to his comfort.

Around noon it strikes me that this is the first day of Dennis's tenure at the hospital that a palliative-team physician has not examined him early in the day as part of their two-rounds-a-day practice. I assume they're waiting until the new care plan can be implemented. I order a breakfast tray: oatmeal, raisin bran, and fruit, plus two cups of tea. As the hours add up and the deep furrows on Dennis's brow seem, against all possibility, to get even deeper, I jettison all attempts to appear patient in my waiting. Dennis can no longer speak, but his involuntary moans evoke my sympathy and fuel my impatience.

I ask Marla if she has had any contact with the palliative MDs—Dr. Ali in particular, whom I had expected to follow up with me this morning. Marla, who had been so precisely attentive earlier in the day, goes vague on me. That's never a good sign. It usually means there's an issue with the reigning MDs. I immediately think of the Other Wife. The medical experience that has become central to my sanity as I play Dennis's cruise director here on the sixteenth floor has given me insight she lacks.

I know something's up here. But would you, Other Wife?

I need to speak with Dr. Ali, so I press a little harder with Marla.

"I saw her earlier..." Marla mutters as she slips out the door. Another hour stretches out, and I ask if Marla would be kind enough to ask Dr. Ali to come in when she has a minute. Marla averts her eyes, adjusts some notation in the electronic record, and leaves again. She's notably less chatty than she was earlier in the day. Perhaps there are medical complications with another of her patients. Is she annoyed that Dennis's room is so far away from her other patient rooms? I know the nursing staff hates that sort of inefficiency. Is it me that annoys Marla? Maybe she doesn't appreciate my active involvement in Dennis's care. Attentive family can be perceived as a complication rather than an asset. Regardless, Marla is my best conduit to Dr. Ali, so I ask again around two thirty.

I hope you don't think you're the only person unable to get the attention you believe you and your beloved need, Other Wife. It's just part of hospital life. Be bold and persistent.

I ask directly, "Are the palliative care people in a meeting all together?"

"Yes," she answers before her information filter can kick in. Flustered by my direct approach, she feigns distraction and leaves again.

It's after five when Dennis and I finally get our audience. Dr. Ali, Dr. Gallagher, and another MD from the ethics committee come into the room together. Their appearance as a united front jangles my nerves. Two of these women know me fairly well—or at least in ways that might garner intimacy. But no smile greets me. No eyes find mine. My breath catches, and my mind races to make sense of the emotional wall that has apparently been erected over the last twenty-four hours. It's an instinctive train of thought, although it's silly to speculate when those who know the answers to my most pressing questions are standing right in front of me. Well, not exactly in front of me. As Dennis slips further from life on earth, I position myself in ways that assure him I am near. At the time of this late-day rendezvous, I'm kneeling on the metal frame of the bed's upper end with my forearms around Dennis's head. The damp washcloth I'm using to coerce his fever down is in my right hand. My left palm cradles the side of his head.

"I am so glad you're here," I admit. "Look at his face. He's still in so much pain." No one says anything. My queries turn to concerns, and now they spill out in something just short of panic. I try to breathe deeply and focus on listening rather than speaking.

"We need to make a change," Dr. Ali starts. "We're going to lower the sedation tonight."

Just short of panic morphs into the real thing.

"But you can see that he's suffering!" It comes out sounding more like the accusation it is than the question I want to feign.

"Susan, I'm sorry, but Dr. Stefanowicz and her department—"

"Oh." It comes to me suddenly. "They think I'm trying to kill him." My upper body whips around to face Dr. Ali from my perch at Dennis's pillow. We lock eyes briefly, and she shakes her head slowly and purposefully.

"Not you. Me." We stare at each other. She has had more time to process this than I have. I wait for her to explain.

Dr. Gallagher steps in to help. "The department feels the need for a full physical assessment and has requested that we lift all sedation so that this can be done tomorrow."

Before my civility can check me, I lash out. *What did you say?* The three MDs in the room are quick to help me turn from my unedifying and ultimately useless tact.

"We don't want to go there," one says, immediately followed by another doctor's promise: "We just want to focus on what we can do for Dennis."

I'm not proud of my outburst and mean it when I apologize. I'm not sure if this is the point when I burst into tears. I think so. I know that I do because I will later get a look at a white-sick face with eye makeup streaking my cheeks like war paint. I neither feel nor apparently look like myself, so defeated and without recourse as I am. For the next thirty minutes or so, the three MDs and I talk around Dennis's bed about what has transpired during the day. The MDs are discreet, and Dr. Gallagher apologizes that I should have to be concerned with hospital politics. But the fact remains that I am, and my husband's dying body is also at their mercy. During the half hour we talk, Dennis's moans serenade us poignantly, and his eyes press shut tighter and tighter. His frown lines slide down his face into his eye sockets and overtake the fever-ruddy rumpled skin like a dirty shirt tossed in a hamper.

Dennis's visible suffering leads Dr. Stein to present a compromise plan. She suggests that the sedation be lowered incrementally. "I would never just stop opiates without tittering down," she asserts.

When there is nothing more to say, Dr. Ali walks around Dennis's bed to the pump that controls the amount of medication coursing through my husband's veins. He moans. With her hand quite literally on the dial, Dr. Ali freezes. "This is wrong, and I'm not going to do it." With that pronouncement, she shoves her hand into the pocket of her lab coat and walks out of the room.

I assume that one of the two remaining MDs will do the deed. They look at one another and then turn to leave. Dr. Gallagher turns back and leans close to my deflated form cradling my husband and advises, "When the specialist comes to do the evaluation, tell them your story."

"They won't believe me," slips out in a voice just above a whisper.

"This must be so discouraging." Dr. Gallagher sympathizes before she leaves. She has left a bit of her heart hovering over Dennis's bed and I guard it through the next few hours as I struggle with the sense that, even with all my professional end-of-life experience, the health care power of attorney that Dennis filled out and discussed so carefully with me, my hospital work, and my undying commitment to advocating for palliative care, it appears that the allopathic medical system will not give my Dennis this one final gift. I am powerless—if not without a voice—in this space. My grief is profound. I cannot imagine my heart breaking any more raggedly.

I inhale deeply and cry proportionately for a while into the pillow that Dennis and I share. Then I get up, intending to use a washcloth to get my game face back on. One look in the mirror makes it clear that a washcloth is not going to do it. I shower and put on clean clothes. I smooth my hair as it dries and put on face powder, lipstick, and eyeliner. Mascara is clearly no match for my emotions. I settle back in a small chair propped up to the side of Dennis's bed and do a moderate back bend so that my head rests lightly on Dennis's rib cage as I wait for a specialist to come and turn off my suffering husband's sedation. I wonder what I will say to the specialist. I wonder what recourse I might invoke. I wonder if perhaps seeing Dennis the way the palliative team has—moaning and grimacing and edematous, and beginning to turn a mottled purple as his circulation slows—they will relent.

I put my nose up to Dennis's and tell him what I think he needs to hear. "Dream Man, it's getting really ugly here. You don't need to stay around and wait for this hospital to give you permission to go. Just get out of here. Go to heaven now, Dream Man. You have done an *amazing* job investing in the girls and me. We will miss you terribly, but we'll be okay. You don't have to stay here for us. Really, Dream. Go.

Go to heaven...And if I fall behind, wait for me." Ever more resigned to the imminence of Dennis's death, I sit back in the little chair and bury my face in his armpit. I just want to get as close as I can and stay there for as long as I can.

Eventually I pry myself away from the only place I ever want to be and wander into the hall. Of all people, I bump into a Catholic priest making his rounds. Perhaps my face gives me away, or maybe priests can sense when someone is torn between heaven and earth, but Father John immediately recognizes my need. He introduces himself and offers to perform the Sacrament of the Sick for Dennis. I agree, and he escorts me back to Dennis's room, where we stand on either side of the bed and each put a hand on each of Dennis's shoulders.

I don't know Father John, and I'm not Roman Catholic, but I know this is an important moment. My first encounter with this priest occurred a few days earlier. I was in one of my trances, intentionally absorbing my husband's final days on earth. I had pulled a small, straight-backed chair to Dennis's left side. My arms were threaded through its side arm and linked around Dennis's neck. My eyes were barely open as I concentrated on the feel of my husband—the essence of him that had pulled me into his aura a quarter century ago. It was in that sacred space and with those slit eyes that I saw an older man push the door to Dennis's hospital room ajar, make the solid, clinical assessment that this was a private moment, and turn on his heels without a word. Sometimes the best ministry is to honor solitude. I knew then that this gentle soul, Father John, would be the one to administer last rites to my husband. My Irish husband, who had been baptized Dennis Patrick Sheehan, received first Holy Communion, penance, and confirmation in the Catholic Church. The only sacrament he received outside of the Church, much to his grandmothers' chagrin, was his holy matrimony to me.

Now I will see to it that his grandmothers would be pleased with this final rite. Father John asks if there is a particular passage from the Bible that I would like read. Dennis was mediating on Psalm 62 during his last weeks. The gentle priest suggests that I read that Psalm aloud. I begin, "My soul finds rest in God alone…" And the rest is a surreal combination of the Lord's Prayer, anointing, and benediction.

Father John turns to leave, but then he hesitates at the door, looks over at me sitting at Dennis's bedside, and offers another sacred grace—his personal blessing. "You know it's okay to get in the bed with him?" I assure him that I do and smile at the sweet irony of a man who has taken a vow of celibacy being used by God to honor a dying marriage.

Roughly three hours later, the door to Dennis's room swings open again. It's not the specialist I'm anticipating, but Dr. Ali. "I pace when I am thinking," she tosses in my direction as she holds firm ground in a room that is thus transformed from Dennis's bedroom to her office. Four steps. Pivot. Turn. Repeat. She watches her feet—even when she speaks. "When did we stop hydration?"

"We never did. We just didn't start it when Dennis lost the ability to swallow and just stopped drinking on Saturday."

Dr. Ali reviews the full week of medication history and clinical responses. She stops a few times to read from the electronic medical record exuding its bruised blue cast on Dennis's world. She stands still. Then she paces again. I stand with my hand on Dennis's elephantine arm and watch his grimace shift and roll like sands blowing on a beach.

"Look," I interject. "I obviously want what is best for Dennis, but this is not worth your license. He is actively dying. This will be over soon, and there are other patients who need you." I'm bracing myself for what appears to be the inevitable.

"This isn't just about Dennis. I need to do what I think is right," Dr. Ali responds.

I'm not entirely sure what she thinks is right. I need to know. So I watch with every sense God had given me and approach her again. "I understand that you've thrown yourself in front of a bus for us, and I am grateful. But I want you to get up before there are any tire tracks on your chest."

That image elicits eye contact from Dr. Ali but no words. More pacing. Then a measured response: "I think the driver got off the bus, but I don't know about tomorrow. I think we should add hydration to avoid any sense that we are contributing to Dennis's decline." I agree to this for political reasons. It's not the best choice for Dennis, since generally, dehydration is a very comfortable way to die. At this point, Dennis's kidneys are shutting down, and the fluids dripping into him with his medication are not being absorbed and eliminated efficiently. His hands and feet began to swell a few days ago. Now his arms and torso protrude from sheets rumpled by vain attempts to find comfort. Those once familiar arms now look and feel like water balloons. I know that adding hydration will likely cause Dennis's skin to begin to weep and tear with little provocation. But we are in a bigger game now, and I know that there need to be concessions on my part.

It's close to 10:00 p.m. by now, and I want to be very clear about with what medication and at what rates Dennis will be treated overnight. When I ask this directly, Dr. Ali seems to look right though me as she says, "The service is off the unit for the night. I have left orders in the chart that no resident or intern is to make changes in the care plan."

"So the Ativan and Fentanyl will keep running at the current rate?"

Like a pull-string doll with only a limited number of responses, she repeats "The service is off the unit for the night."

I need to know how to work with the nurse during the night. I attempt to verify that Dennis will also be entitled to additional medication, called a "bolus" in medical lingo, for the breakthrough pain that seems especially distressing to him. "And the bolus is still available through the night?" I beg.

Again, the only response I get is, "The service is off the unit for the night." Dr. Ali takes another look into the blue monitor's haze. She puts a hand self-consciously on my shoulder and pauses. Without a word, she pivots and strides right out the door. We both know that she will think of little else as she finds her way home and goes through the motions of her own private life. We both know that the next day might be grueling politically. While our bodies are running out of energy, the ethical hairs on the back of our necks are standing on end. For different reasons and in different ways, Dr. Ali and I have made a pact to do as close to our understanding of "right" as we are able.

Fast-forward a few weeks. The summer skies hang low and dark outside the well-appointed conference room where I sit with the chief medical officer (CMO) and the director of quality strategies. The CMO rehearses details of Dennis's care over the eleven-day hospitalization. He speaks methodically in an even, measured tone, unimpeded by my periodic interruptions. I think I know the facts since I rarely left the room. I slept little. The facts I know warrant the audience I am being offered on this day. When the CMO cites data I believe to be erroneous, I am eager to correct. Three or four times he repeats the data in his version, and I interject mine. There is no evidence that he hears me. He doesn't seem to want clarification. His speech becomes slightly pressured. He continues until he's out of wind and then sucks in as much air as his lungs can hold. He looks at me and informs me that there are elements of Dennis's care that have been identified as "sentinel" events. He holds the lock on my eyes. Does he suspect that I know the implications of that word? Is he sure that I don't? The walls seem to close in around me as I suck in whatever air is still left in that room.

I know what a sentinel event means to a health care provider. It means that, according to The Joint Commission, a nonprofit that oversees quality controls in US health care, there has been an error noted which either did lead or could have led to significantly negative patient outcomes. There's a formal process initiated by the identification of a sentinel event. It represents both an opportunity to learn and an opening for litigation. The latter invariably informs subsequent interaction with families. I'm suddenly aware that I am being handled. I'm a threat to be mitigated and a potentially huge litigation to be avoided. And all along I thought I was just the wife.

TALKING POINTS FOR MORTALS

1. In your mind, what events in your medical history stand out as worthy of special investigation?
2. Have you found your loved ones to be concerned with these same things?
3. What might you do to encourage this investigation by your treatment team?

■ ■ ■

CHAPTER 12

Autopsy

[aw-top-see] n. medical procedure during which a dead body is reduced for analysis of proximal cause of death and contributing physical realities

> *My e-mailing post is made from home at 5:17 a.m.:*
> *"Dennis died peacefully—FINALLY—by the grace of God and the mercy of the Northwestern Memorial Hospital's palliative team. We are sad. We are relieved. We know that Dennis is at this minute rejoicing with the angels in his glorified body. That should cover us for at least some of the obvious that is not so good...like what to do next. I put in some laundry. I called our daughters and my father-in-law. I put out the recycling. Life will just keep happening, and by God's grace that will be a very good thing."*
> *What does that life mean for you, grieving Other Wife? I wonder how I might help you.*

I somehow miss Dennis's death although I am physically present. I will have little memory of the events of the hour in which my husband actually, officially, pronounced-by-the-house-doc dies. That will be 1:45 a.m. on this June morning in 2008. Of course, the actual time of death is before that. House MDs do not stand around waiting to witness the moment of death; rather, the nurses call them after the fact. By the time he comes, I will be standing at the foot of the bed watching. My hand will be spread around Dennis's right foot, my fingers parrying with his toes. I will notice his high instep. I will notice that Dennis's nails still need a clipping that they will never get. I will be both wrung dry from exhaustion and wrapped tight in adrenaline. I will not cry, and I will think that is odd.

A couple of hours ago, I had curled up in the room to try to sleep a little. Around midnight, the young nurse assigned to Dennis for the first time, Melanie Sparks, leaned over me to say, "His breathing is changing." In fact, it had been increasingly labored for days. Dennis's lungs were congested by what we all suspect and the autopsy will prove: Dennis had aspiration pneumonia, which is a serious infection that can run right through a weakened body. Dennis's body certainly counted as weakened. Every breath makes odd sounds. My husband rattled and wheezed and crackled, except when he stopped breathing completely for increasingly large proportions of minutes. Then he heaved and started the chorus again. Tonight what Melanie meant is that the breaths are of a pattern known as Cheyenne Stokes, typical of the last hours of life.

I climbed into that oversized bed designed to protect Dennis's now fragile skin but big enough for two of us. I just lay beside him and ravenously collected my last bundle of the parts of him that could be gathered. I traced the edges of his face and ears and neck and marveled at this man and all he meant to me. When my eyes move to his arm resting on a wadded-up pillow, I marveled equally at how that man who means so much to me was disappearing. His arms are puffy and pale; the crook at the inside of his elbow was unfamiliar to me. What I had always affectionately called his "Irish potato-picker hands"—square and strong working hands—are mottled like a bluish marble and badly swollen. I am saying good-bye. Still and again and forever. By the time that house MD arrives, I am clear that I do not begrudge Dennis his hard-earned death.

In the midst of this fog, I have enough of the instinctive health care advocate in me to respond to the perfunctory offer of an autopsy. "Yes, please," I hear myself saying. "I would appreciate that." This from a woman who had earlier no inclination to prove a known reality of no consequence! In the past few days there has been unfathomable drama. The specialists have threatened legal action against the palliative care team on the grounds that end-of-life treatment is precluded by protocol and law unless it is summarily verified. Their opinion is that this has not been done. My opinion, and that of other MDs, differs. In the middle of the night, while Dennis's body is still warm and I am packing our belongings and fingering his wedding band—which is awkwardly held hostage around my own ringed finger—I remember the hospital politics. That should not be something of which I am proud. That should not have been at all.

The phrase "*Hie locus est ubi mors gaudet succurrete*" is hung in many pathology labs. It is Latin for what is acknowledged to the rest of us in English: "This is the place where death rejoices to help those who live." An autopsy and its subsequent report, by definition, do nothing to help the person being examined. An autopsy is all about learning lessons that will impact the lives of others. It is a precious gift that costs at once nothing at all and more than anyone would ever elect to offer.

I am certain that Dennis's autopsy will show nothing other than the sad ravages of his diagnosed disease having progressed in linear if alarmingly geometric rate. There will be typical end-of-life notations: aspiration pneumonia, common when people are weak and are not able to adequately protect their airways by coughing or otherwise clearing secretions. I expect significant weight loss to be noted. I expect some thrush to be evident in his mouth and upper GI tract. I can visually assess the decubiti that erupted on skin once smooth. So smooth in fact that it was resistant to mosquito bites and poison ivy and kitchen burns and various other signs of life that plagued the rest of us. Now his skin has failed him too, in sync with the rest of his physical body shutting down: coma sores, thrush, bed sores as deep as a stage three (maximum is four), and hives and rashes of various description and etiology erupting with a life that seemed to feed off Dennis's death.

A kind nursing aide helps me load a metal cart with our personal supplies—half a bottle of red wine, some fruit, that shaving kit that I have been appropriating as my own, Dennis's iPod and Bible, the dirty laundry we have accumulated, and a couple of boxers and T-shirts that could have kept me here for another couple days before I would have needed to venture out for supplies. There is Dennis's leg brace. There is the now battered cane that a dear group of friends presented to him when it was clear that walking unaided was no longer a safe option. There is the walker that Dennis was too weak to use and the gait belt that helped him stretch when his body spasms needed some counter force. There is his pillow and case, damp with the effort of dying. There is the bell curve of my statistical outlier on the wall; I carefully peel it off and tuck it in a book. All of this is loaded onto that cart or over my shoulders, into the elevator, and out into the soft predawn city morning. My car, which has not been moved in ten days, has a flat tire, but the man in the garage pumps it up for me. I pray that, even without a patch, my car with my husband's last serviceable belongings will travel the thirty miles home before it deflates again. It does.

In that morning, so early that the sky still thinks it is night, I drive home and make three phone calls. I call our firstborn, who is cocooned with friends in Massachusetts. Brittany will begin her remarks at her dad's memorial service with the words, "It's no secret that I have always been a daddy's girl." Indeed it is not, and while she and I both knew that one day I would be calling to tell her that her dad had died, it breaks my own heart anew. I am an adult with forty-seven years of life to ready me for this day. Brittany is a twenty-two-year-old freshly minted college graduate who has always greeted her world with her dad's exuberance. This is the first day that she will not also have his steadying hand. My call has woken her, but it is the loss that she feels all the way to her feet that makes the few words she utters sound hollow.

Juliana answers her phone more quickly. That night owl seems to pull courage from some well within as she asks a few clarifying questions and then, kindly, "Mom, are you okay?"

"Yes, Boo, I am okay, but I think that we are going to miss Dad forever."

The girls have been privy to the precipitous decline that their dad had experienced during the hospitalization. They are also my girls, and we have shared the past two decades fairly intimately. Calling them is my heart's first priority. Calling Dennis's father is a charge that somehow I feel less well equipped to execute. I decide to wait until five thirty, which would be six-thirty for him on the east coast. He typically rises early. I think a great deal about my script, but when he picks up the phone and speaks through the cobwebs, I hear myself say quite simply, "Dad? It's Susan. Dad? We lost Dennis this morning. I am so sorry." My script was more poetic and less direct.

"Oh…my. Ah." These are not words. These are the falling shards of a parent's love. In those shards I can hear my father-in-law's box of bits of his third child: ice cream on the beach, a white first communion suit, Little League games, Troop 39, divergent politics, and the calls after every Giants game in recent years. "I am so sorry, Susan," he chokes out. I know that he is more sorry than I will ever fully understand. I offer the logistics of visitation and memorial service. I hear the labored breathing of a man who has just learned that his fifty-two-year-old son is dead. We say good-bye. After cradling the phone for a minute or so, I burst into tears for the first of many post-mortem Dennis laments.

Later that day, my father-in-law calls and leaves a message on my voice mail. He is wondering about an obituary in the local paper of Dennis's hometown in New Jersey. He begins, "Susan? Uh, this is Da—um, Jack…er, John Sheehan." And again I burst into tears at the vulnerability of this big, strong man who in one day has lost his son and—he seems to fear—his rightful connection to his two granddaughters and me. I regroup and find a little bit of joy in this surreal day by calling back and telling my husband's father that in the last twenty-five years, I have gotten used to "Dad," and I planned to keep using that appellation. That happens in the same minute that I resolve that my girls and I will spend our first post-Dennis Thanksgiving with the Sheehan clan.

Without any possibility of changing the course of my husband's dying days, my attention turns quickly to the task of somehow supporting the Other Wife who has been my intimate companion.

I cannot do nothing in the wake of the 10 days that I have just experienced or perhaps better stated the course of Dennis' disease plus 10 days. I write a letter of suggestions for better patient care to each and every MD in the hospital directory of the appropriate department. I am beginning my work to give a human face to what might otherwise be a sterile and distant presentation of raw data. I feel the raw part. The data alone reveals too little about real people and their real struggles. I will continue to press for dialogue. I will continue to press not only because my husband's face is etched on my heart but also because there are countless other faces shadowing my mind. The most compelling and propelling to me is yours, dear Other Wife.

Two months later I am given the final autopsy report, and even then it is not complete. It is noted that "brain (l,650 g) and spinal cord to be examined by neuropathologist after fixation. Results will be issued as an addendum." To me the whole thing is an addendum. The autopsy trails after a rugged hospitalization, which is the culmination of three years of extraordinary suffering. All of it, so stark to me right now, has very little to do with the life of my Dream Man. I sit typing in the room that was originally Dennis's study. He thought the name "office" too heavy for a space that was his delight. It is walled with books. Most have long been our books. There are some that are definitely Dennis's volumes: baseball, US history, and an ancient fifty-two-volume set of Bible exposition that he bought to my chagrin a week before our wedding. The photographs tucked on the shelves are all of Dennis doing real life: sitting on an upturned bucket on the beach, playing in the yard with our kids, and looking over Soldier Field from the press box where he had the delightful privilege of being a field reporter for ESPN during a few Bears games. It is into this space that pages of Dennis's autopsy report spill disordered from my laptop via the printer and onto the floor. Mine is the task of picking up and imposing order on what is so intensely chaotic. Perhaps in this ordering I can eke out more meaning in the way in which my husband left the life he lived so passionately.

The autopsy reduced Dennis's last ten days fairly neatly. "The body is that of a thin, white male who appears older than the stated age of fifty-two years. Patient complained of intractable pain that was unresponsive to multiple treatment modalities...Patient's time of death was 0145..." The report systematically highlights every organ. There are more than you would think; who considers the state of their urethra, parathyroid, thymus, bile ducts, calvarium, and meninges? Mostly the pathologists conclude under each heading that "Microscopic examination...is unremarkable." I want to talk to those pathologists. I irrationally want to explain how that man will be remembered by his family and friends. I cannot help but insert my own autopsy into the framework of these well-trained scientists. It includes things like:

- BONE: remarkable for its ability to lift an average-sized woman high over crowds on South Avenue to see the Christmas display in the Saks windows
- PHARYNX: remarkable for the range of tone it can produce and the people charmed by its crooning
- LUNGS: remarkable for their ability to support a pre-dawn run with simultaneous political commentary
- HEART: remarkable for its ability to beat with others and to extend grace—very, very big

- **STOMACH:** remarkable for its fifty-two-year daily ingestion of obscene quantities of Cheerios and black coffee and disproportionate loads of tuna salad and raisins (not usually together)

I want to tell those MDs that everything about my husband is in fact very remarkable. I want the whole world to know that Dennis Patrick Sheehan cannot be reduced to organs excised from a corpse and evaluated by a microscope in a lab.

TALKING POINTS FOR MORTALS

1. What questions remain unanswered around your medical situation? Do you need those answers? Does someone you love need those answers?

2. From whom will you request support in gathering data toward answering those questions? Do you need those answers to move forward?

■ ■ ■

AFTERWARD

Eulogy

[yoo-luh-jee] n. formal praise of a life well lived and a love lost

Dennis's death is behind me. The focus has turned from his horrific end-of-life drama to the extraordinary man who got lost in the disease, its progression, and various elements of its treatment. I have the privilege of looking back to a time before that wretched season and seeing the man I married. It is such a lovely grace to read and reread an impressive collection of words from people who knew Dennis. Dennis's simple presence calmed others. Dennis's gallant manner charmed them. Dennis's quirky wit entertained everyone. Dennis's open suffering inspired those who, sadly, never knew the other parts. As passionately independent as I have always been, I will never stop being fiercely proud of the privilege of being Mrs. Dennis Patrick Sheehan. Never.

How sad it would be for you to read of these last, difficult days of my husband's life without understanding why this introverted, if verbal, woman would take on a large US teaching hospital to lobby for the best possible care—and then write about it for you. I would tell you that I believe that every person is entitled to such care. I want to introduce myself to you, to tell you what I know and help you find whatever else you might realize you need. I am almost as committed to you, Other Wife, as I have been to my husband. And I want to be for you the steadying force that Dennis continues to be for me. I hear phrases that he used to shower on me and I pass them to you:

Take care of yourself.

The people in this world are so blessed to know you!

You are stronger than you know.

Now I play the soundtracks that are etched in my mind. I want you to be able to play them too. I let them turn slowly. I search for nuance. I play some segments mind-numbingly often. At those times, mind numbing is the goal. Other times my mind flashes sharp, and I recognize myself in the mirror and yield to the reality that this post physical death time is not just a season to survive, but a life to live. I have stopped doing maladaptive things like eating out of containers standing in front of the open fridge and refusing to answer the telephone.

Our twenty-fifth wedding anniversary comes two months after Dennis's death. I consider it our last date. I kick off my shoes in my bed-and-breakfast staging room on the Jersey shore. I look at the plastic bag on the bed. It is thick enough to be almost opaque. There is no chance of it breaking without a sharp cut. I guess cremation services know that their packages must not spill until the time is right. I use nail scissors to pry off the white, cinched closure. I finger the dark, metal, circular identification tag engraved with the facility name and the numbers 6-1-3-0. I cry, at once grateful that there will be some token to bring back to Chicago and struck by the reduction of my husband to six and a half pounds of ashes in a plastic bag, with four digits on an inexpensive piece of metal, engraved unevenly as if by an ancient manual typewriter. The ashes at church forty days before Easter are different from these. At mass the ashes are dark and soft and ceremonial and somehow right as they trace a cross on my forehead. Those ashes always center me. Those ashes remind me of who I am "in Christ Jesus," as the Bible says and the priest reminds. Dennis's ashes are coarse and angular and lightened by bone fragments. When I dip my fingers into them, no satisfying residue clings to me. I put the open bag to my face, but there is nothing fragrant. Wanting so badly to satisfy my soul with a visceral sense of Dennis, I put a tiny bit of charred remains formerly known as my husband on my tongue. It has no taste. I swallow. It is gritty. I like the idea of Dennis being part of my DNA. I decide that I will never tell anyone about my tasting those ashes. The next day I do.

Barefoot and wearing a simple gray shift, I walk across Ocean Avenue. I pad along the boardwalk looking for "our" jetty. Twenty-six years ago Dennis and I made a similar trip to the Jersey shore, and he would later tell me that it was on that jetty, "looking into your big, green eyes," that he decided to marry me. Never mind that it was so dark that night as we made our way over the rocks protruding into the Atlantic Ocean that it is highly unlikely Dennis could have found my eye sockets, much less get lost in their color. He loved to tell me that story, and he stuck by it in the face of all my reason.

As I move from the boardwalk to the sand, the weight of what I have come to do washes over my whole being. The ocean licks the bag that I've been holding at my side. I draw it up against my chest with both arms and walk into the surf, at first teary, then crying, and then something just this side of hysterical. I have forgotten how powerfully loud the ocean is and how the spray snaps off the beach into my face. I am so grateful for the privacy these realities create for me. I press into that surf clutching my precious load. As much as I know that this is precisely what Dennis wanted, and as much as I believe that the ashes are more a symbol of Dennis than anything else, I scream to God that I do not want to surrender them to the dark, undulating expanse I have flown halfway across the country to greet. The waters slam against my legs. After a while, calmer, I decide to pour out just a little bit. By the light of the moon, the ash is discernible in the arc I fling, and discernible until the water snatches it. I walk along the shore making broad arcs with my husband as if we were on a dance floor. I cry until the bag is empty. Somehow it is as if the contents of that bag and my heart are artfully synchronized.

I monitor my steps and note markers to share with our girls and Dennis's family: Bradley Beach off the jetty just north of Second Avenue in Avon-by-the-Sea. I still have the bag. Empty. The first large trash can I see is boldly labeled garbage only. Obviously Dennis's bag is not going there. The next one is labeled recycling. That is the right place, and into that can I carefully set the bag. I linger a moment pondering the word "recycle."

Acknowledgements

This book is a dream come true for me - writing what others would read! - and one that was first envisioned by my husband, Dennis, who had no idea it would be about his death. His sister, Kate Sheehan Roach, grabbed the dream and stoked it in ways too numerous to itemize but most importantly never letting me forget how important its message would be to the Other Wife.

I also want to thank my daughters, Brittany Eleanor and Juliana Purcell whose own precious lives are inevitably woven into this story. They graciously agreed to let those lives be shared on these pages although the memories are mine alone.

Susan E. Sheehan, LCSW, MPA, CT, ACHP-SW is Principal at Finishing Well Consulting LLC. She has graduate degrees in Public Administration, Systems Theory, and Medical Social Work. Her career focus is medical, palliative and hospice social work and in this capacity she has worked with over 2,000 families. She lives in the Chicago area with two lively dogs and has two unleashed adult daughters.

Susan would be delighted to continue to engage you in Talking Points for Mortals through her blog or in her capacity as a consultant.
https://finishingwellconsulting.com